FOOD FACTS

for pregnancy

and breastfeeding

 The National Childbirth Trust

Thank you

Fiona Ford of the University of Sheffield Sainsbury's/
WellBeing 'Eating for Pregnancy' telephone helpline
(0845 130 3646) helped us to update the information in
this book.

Funds towards this publication have been kindly donated
by the Cardiff and Caerphilly branch of the National
Childbirth Trust.

The National Childbirth Trust wants all parents to
have an experience of pregnancy, birth and early
parenthood that enriches their lives and gives them
confidence in being a parent.

For more information about the NCT, see page 209.

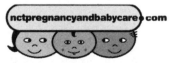

Cover design
Tim McPhee, Book Production Consultants plc

Cover photograph
John Lamb/Getty Images
www.gettyimages.co.uk

FOOD FACTS

for pregnancy

and breastfeeding

**Hannah Hulme Hunter
and Rosemary Dodds**

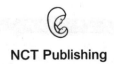

NCT Publishing

First published in 1998 as *The NCT Book of Safe Foods* by
Thorsons/NCT Publishing

© NCT Publishing 2003

Hannah Hulme Hunter and Rosemary Dodds assert the moral right to
be identified as the authors of this work

A catalogue record for this book
is available from the British Library

ISBN 0-9543018-1-1

Printed and bound in the UK by Biddles Ltd

This edition published in 2003 by
NCT Publishing
25-27 High Street
Chesterton
Cambridge
CB4 1ND
www.nctpublishing.co.uk

Contents

About the authors

Rosie Dodds trained as a nutritionist and worked as a research dietitian for nine years. The birth and breastfeeding of her son led her to train as a breastfeeding counsellor with the NCT. In 1993, she joined the charity as Policy Research Officer. In this role she enjoys campaigning and gleaning research on all issues related to feeding.

Hannah Hulme Hunter is a practising midwife. She worked for a time for MIDIRS (Midwives' Information and Resource Service) and also as an NCT breastfeeding counsellor. She has written for many midwifery and parenting journals and practises as a midwife in a maternity unit near Oxford. She has three young children.

Introduction

Eating a balanced diet is perhaps the single most important contribution we can make to our own wellbeing.

During pregnancy you are sharing your food and drink with your unborn baby. You are responsible for her growth and healthy development, as well as your own wellbeing. A good eating pattern during pregnancy: helps your body cope with the special demands of being pregnant; has a positive influence on the future health of your baby; builds up stores of energy and nutrients for times of need; and prepares your body for breastfeeding and nurturing your baby.

But it may not be easy during pregnancy to change your eating habits. Pregnancy is a very busy time for many women – working, looking after a home and family and fitting in clinic appointments. At the same time, you may not be feeling well – you may have pregnancy sickness or tiredness, and you may feel uncomfortably full and big. You may worry about putting on too much weight – or about not putting on enough. Many women are concerned about food safety – there seem to be so many rules and warnings about paté and eggs and soft cheeses. Sometimes it just seems easier to open another packet of chocolate biscuits! And so we decided to write this book.

The information in this book is based on sound scientific research. If the findings of the research are unclear, we say so. We offer you clear and unbiased information – but we do not make decisions for you. Each woman reading this will have her own needs and priorities, and you alone can make the decisions that suit your life. Only when risks are clear-cut do we firmly state a recommended course of action.

Whether you are planning to get pregnant, have just discovered you're pregnant or you are due to have your baby next month, we hope that this book will guide you, ease some of your anxieties – and support you when you decide what to buy, cook and eat during pregnancy. Above all, we hope this book will help make eating fun.

Hannah Hulme Hunter
Rosemary Dodds
February 2003

New research studies, discovering the effects of certain foods and drinks on mother and child during pregnancy and while breastfeeding, are being published all the time. Theses studies are widely publicised in the national press and it is up to all of us to stay as well informed as possible. To the best of our knowledge, all the information in this book is correct at time of going to press.

1

What is 'healthy eating'?

Healthy eating is about choosing a balance of food, and feeling your best physically and mentally. Healthy eating is about real food – and enjoying eating.

In this chapter we describe the main food groups, explain why they are important and talk about the part that each group plays in a healthy and balanced diet.

Getting the balance right

Imagine an empty plate. Mentally divide the plate into three.

One-third will be full of energy foods: the starchy carbohydrates – pasta, potatoes, rice, yam, bread or cereals. Another third will be packed with fruit and vegetables. Divide the remaining third of the plate into three unequal sections, one a lot smaller than the other two. One of these sections is for protein foods, needed for growth and repair of our bodies – meat, fish, nuts, cooked beans and so on. The other section is for dairy products: the milk-based foods, rich in calcium and other minerals – fresh milk, yoghurt, cheese. The tiny bit in the middle is for fatty and sugary foods.

Now put some food onto your plate. Fill one whole third with rice, potatoes or pasta. Pack another third with lightly cooked vegetables. Put a small portion of fish or lean meat in one of the remaining bigger bits. In the other, put a tub of plain yoghurt. In the tiny bit in the middle, put a teaspoonful of honey to mix into the yoghurt. Pour yourself a glass or two of water. There – a balanced meal!

What about breakfast? Fill one-third of your plate with tinned grapefruit segments. Fill the next third with 2–3 slices of wholemeal toast. If you want to (and it doesn't matter if you don't for one meal), add an egg or a slice of lean ham. Place a glass of semi-skimmed milk in one of the smaller sections, and a pat of butter for the toast in the tiny one in the middle. Another balanced meal.

A quick working lunch? Fill one-third of your plate with a large roll of wholemeal bread. Pack the next third with some well-washed salad leaves, a sliced tomato and a crisp, green apple. In the small protein section put a hard-boiled egg or some slices of tasty Cheddar. (Don't worry about the milk section; the cheese has taken care of that one this time.) Spread the bread roll with a small knob of low-fat spread, and wash down your meal with a carton of unsweetened orange juice.

Treats

Some women find it more helpful to imagine the plate filled with food for the whole day – or even for several days. So long as we get the balance right over about a week, that's OK. This means that the bag of crisps we couldn't resist in the cinema can fill up the tiny fatty foods section for several days – provided we don't try to squeeze in extra dollops of cream as well! And the second helping of roast lamb enjoyed at the weekend can take care of our protein needs for a while, too.

But beware: many foods overlap the sections on the plate and need to be counted into both. Streaky bacon, for example, and ham with the fat still attached, will fill the small protein section – and overlap into the tiny fat section. (So no extra butter or spread for that meal.) Likewise, breakfast cereals are an excellent way of filling the carbohydrate section, but if they contain added sugar, that's the sugar section overflowing as well. This is why it's a good idea to choose low-fat and low-sugar foods – and leave the fat and sugar section free for the odd sweet or bag of crisps or whatever other treats we fancy.

Food choices from across the world

Wherever you come from, and whatever the origins of your choice of food, you can use these guidelines for a balanced diet. Simply decide in which group the foods you enjoy belong, and plan your meals around the same proportions described above.

In fact, we can all learn a lot about balanced eating from the food of other countries. Most Indian meals are based on plenty of rice or chapati, a vegetable curry and occasional fish or eggs. Traditional Italian meals generally involve lots of pasta, tasty tomato or milk-based sauces and perhaps a small quantity of meat. Much Chinese cooking centres on stir-fries of noodles, lightly cooked vegetables and seafood. Many traditional African meals involve plenty of starchy carbohydrate – yam, maybe, or pounded cassava – a spicy stew and green leafy vegetables.

Just one word of caution: if you also enjoy fatty foods such as chips, pies and crisps, keep a close eye on the total amount of fat in your diet.

Now let's look more closely at the foods in each section of our plate.

What is a nutrient?

A nutrient is any substance that gives us nourishment and contributes to the smooth working of our bodies.

What are carbohydrates?

A third of our plate is packed with starchy carbohydrate foods. Carbohydrates should be the main food group that give us energy (calories). We all need energy foods, simply to keep our bodies working well. Some of us need more energy than others; a farmer, active all day in the open air, will need more energy than a secretary sitting at a desk. But even sitting and thinking uses up energy!

Caring for young children and running a home is particularly demanding work. An adequate intake of energy foods is very important, not only to give us the strength to keep going but to help us feel enthusiastic and happy doing so. During late pregnancy you need slightly more energy than at other times – but not much! It is certainly not true that you need to 'eat for two'. We talk more about this in Chapter 5.

There are two types of carbohydrates – starches and sugars.

Starchy carbohydrates

Starchy foods include things like breakfast cereals, bread, chapati, nan, pitta, rice, pasta, noodles, potatoes, yam and plantain. These foods tend to be good and filling. The energy from starchy foods is slowly converted into sugars and gradually absorbed by our bodies. This means we feel satisfied for longer.

Starchy carbohydrate foods give us more than just energy. They are also important sources of other valuable nutrients – protein, vitamins, minerals and fibre. Starchy carbohydrate foods tend to be fairly cheap to buy.

Sugary carbohydrates

Sugary carbohydrates are found in foods such as sweet biscuits, cakes, jellies, puddings and sweets. These foods are not very filling and they can be expensive to buy. Sugary carbohydrates give us a quick boost of energy, but this energy is only short-lasting so we are likely to feel hungry again soon afterwards.

Sugary carbohydrates have very little nutritional value. This is why it is best not to eat too many sugary foods. It is far better to eat plenty of the starchy carbohydrate foods mentioned above – foods that give us more than just energy. We talk more about sugary foods a little later in this chapter.

Wholemeal foods

Generally, wholemeal or brown varieties of rice, pasta, cereals and bread tend to contain more vitamins, minerals and fibre than the refined or white kinds. For example, wholemeal bread contains half as much again of some of the important B group of vitamins than the same amount of white bread – and twice as much fibre. Wholemeal foods are very useful during pregnancy, when sometimes you may not feel like eating much, because even a relatively small quantity of a wholemeal food will still give you plenty of energy and other nutrients.

Wholemeal breakfast cereals are especially good value in nutritional terms. All breakfast cereals are good energy foods, and most are fortified. (Fortified means that extra vitamins or iron have been added.) Wholemeal cereals are also particularly rich in fibre. Add milk, maybe a few pieces of fresh or tinned fruit, and you have a balanced, get-up-and-go breakfast. Many people enjoy breakfast cereals at other times of the day, too.

How much starchy carbohydrate?

Along with fruit and vegetables, starchy carbohydrates make up the bulk of a balanced diet. Try to include some starchy foods in each meal – and aim for a total of six servings throughout the day. A 'serving' of starchy carbohydrates is equivalent to:

- ❏ 2 large slices of bread
- ❏ 1 large bread roll, a pitta or a nan
- ❏ 2 Weetabix
- ❏ a large bowl of breakfast cereal 'flakes'
- ❏ a large bowl of porridge
- ❏ 2 fist-sized potatoes or 2 pieces of yam
- ❏ a portion (about 6 tablespoons) of cooked pasta
- ❏ a portion (about 4 heaped tablespoons) of rice

What are minerals?

Minerals are inorganic (not living) nutrients found naturally in many foods. Iron, calcium and zinc are examples of important minerals. Minerals are necessary for many body functions, including control of the balance of fluids in our bodies, as well as strong bones and teeth. As with vitamins, it is best to get minerals from our food, rather than take supplements.

What are vitamins?

Vitamins are special substances that our bodies need in order to function normally. Vitamins occur naturally in many foods – but no single food contains all vitamins except breastmilk. Only one vitamin (vitamin D) can be made within our bodies – most have to be obtained from our food. Some vitamins can be stored in our bodies while others need to be eaten each day. We only need very small amounts of each vitamin. It is best to get vitamins from our food, rather than from supplements (except for folic acid). Too much vitamin A can be harmful during pregnancy.

Why are vegetables and fruit so important?

The next third of our plate is filled with vegetables and fruit. These foods are bursting with valuable nutrients including vitamins (especially vitamin C and folic acid) and minerals. Fruit and vegetables are our main source of antioxidants – special chemicals found naturally in foods that help protect our bodies against heart disease, cancer and the effects of pollution.

Fruit and vegetables are also a good source of fibre. Fibre (also found in cereals) is the part of our food that is not digested by our bodies. It passes through our digestive system and makes up the bulk of our faeces (bowel motion or poo). Fibre plays an important part in keeping our digestive systems running smoothly and preventing bowel diseases. If we do not have enough fibre in our diet, we may become constipated (have difficulty in passing a bowel motion).

Shopping for fruit and vegetables

If you can, buy fresh fruit and vegetables. Green leafy vegetables are good sources of folic acid. Yellow fruit such as mangoes and apricots, and citrus fruits such as oranges and grapefruits, are rich in vitamin C. But the main thing is to choose fruit and vegetables that you enjoy – and eat plenty!

Try to choose clean, undamaged items, store in a cool place and wash them well at home. Fruit and vegetables sold loose tend to be cheaper than trimmed and packaged items. Some market stall holders and green grocers sell their produce off at reduced prices at the end of the shopping day. Eat fruit and vegetables within a few days, while they are still fresh. And remember that over-cooking of vegetables will greatly reduce their vitamin content – and spoil their taste.

How much vegetables and fruit?

We cannot eat too much fruit and too many vegetables! We should all aim to eat five servings each day. A serving of fruit and vegetables is equivalent to:

❑ a piece of fruit – one apple, a single banana, a large slice of melon and so on
❑ 12 chunks of tinned pineapple
❑ a small glass of unsweetened fruit juice
❑ a large bowl of salad
❑ a large tomato
❑ 3 tablespoons of peas
❑ 2 tablespoons of carrots or cabbage
❑ a handful of raisins
❑ vegetable curry or vegetable stir-fry (counts as two servings if eaten as a main meal)

What about protein?

Protein foods fit into one of the smaller sections of our plate. This may surprise some people. The traditional approach to English meal planning tended to over-emphasise our need for protein – especially for meat protein. Nutritionists now know that we do not need as much protein as previously thought.

But protein is still a very important part of our diet. We need it to repair and maintain the basic building blocks of our bodies – our cells. We also need it to grow new cells; in particular, we need protein while pregnant to grow our babies. We need protein, too, to grow new blood cells and to produce antibodies (the special cells that help our bodies fight infection). Meat protein, in particular, is rich in valuable minerals such as iron and zinc. We talk more about these nutrients in Chapter 2.

Protein comes from two food sources – animal and vegetable. Whatever the source, the basic component of protein is the amino acid. There are many different amino acids. Our bodies can make some, but most need to be taken in our diet. The balance of amino acids in animal protein (in meat, milk and eggs) is similar to the balance required by our bodies. The balance of amino acids in vegetable protein (in nuts and lentils, for example) varies from food to food. This is why people who do not eat meat or drink milk need to eat a wide range of vegetable protein in order to get a good balance of amino acids.

Pregnancy increases the need for protein – but only by a small amount. A balanced diet including 2–3 servings of protein – vegetable, meat or a mixture of both – will easily take care of the extra bit required during pregnancy.

Animal protein

Animal sources of protein include all kinds of meat and fish. Turkey, chicken and fish tend to contain less saturated fat than red meat. (Saturated fat is the most harmful type of fat.) So, if you eat red meat (such as beef, lamb and pork), try to choose lean cuts – remember, you don't need much!

Oily fish, such as mackerel, tuna and sardines (fresh or tinned), are useful sources of protein – because they also give us essential fatty acids. We explain more about fatty acids later in this chapter.

Vegetable protein

Vegetable sources of protein include:

❑ nuts and seeds
❑ peanut butter (peanuts contain as much protein as most cheeses and twice as much as eggs – but see the note about peanut allergy at the end of Chapter 7)
❑ meat substitutes, tofu (made from soya beans) and Quorn (made from a fungus)
❑ pulses including lentils (such as masur dhal), baked beans, kidney beans, black-eyed beans, butter beans, borlotti beans, mung beans, broad beans and all kinds of peas.

A well-planned vegetarian diet is extremely healthy. Vegetable protein foods are rich in fibre as well as protein, and contain many vitamins and minerals. Avoiding meat and using vegetable protein foods can be a good way of reducing your intake of saturated fat, and increasing your intake of fibre.

The protein in vegetable protein foods is less concentrated than the protein in animal protein foods. Servings tend to be larger. If you do not eat meat or drink milk, it is a good idea to include a serving of vegetable protein at each meal. Some other important nutrients are less concentrated in vegetable protein. Choose vegetable protein foods rich in iron, zinc, calcium and vitamin B_{12} (more about all of these nutrients in Chapter 2).

How much animal protein?

We can get enough protein from just two servings of meat protein foods each day. A serving of animal protein is equivalent to:

- ❏ 2 slices of roast chicken or turkey
- ❏ half a small mackerel fillet
- ❏ 2 rounded tablespoons of tinned tuna chunks
- ❏ 1 small fillet of white fish such as cod
- ❏ 2 slices of lamb, beef or pork
- ❏ 1 small lamb or pork chop
- ❏ 2 eggs
- ❏ 1 slice of tinned corned beef

How much vegetable protein?

Aim for 2–3 servings of vegetable protein foods each day. A serving of vegetable protein is equivalent to:

- ❑ 1 tablespoon of peanut butter
- ❑ 2 heaped tablespoons of nuts or seeds
- ❑ 3 tablespoonfuls of cooked kidney beans or chick-peas
- ❑ one-third of a large tin (420g) of baked beans
- ❑ 2–3 tablespoons of thick lentil dhal
- ❑ a small pot (100g) of hummus (try the low-fat variety)
- ❑ a large cup of soya milk
- ❑ one-third of a packet of tofu

What about milk foods?

The second of the small sections on our imaginary plate is for milk-based foods, or dairy products. Milk – and foods made from it, such as cheese, yoghurt and fromage frais – is an excellent and convenient source of calcium, zinc, some B group vitamins and protein.

Milk and milk products contain varying amounts of fat, depending on the type of milk and the way in which it has been processed. 'Skimmed' milk has had all the fat removed and 'semi-skimmed' milk has had half the fat removed. Both have the same amount of protein as whole milk – and slightly more calcium.

Liquid milk also contains plenty of water, so a glass of chilled, semi-skimmed milk is a refreshing and nutritious drink. If you do not like the taste of milk, try flavouring it with mashed banana or pulped mango. Use unsweetened cocoa powder in hot milk for a comforting evening drink.

The calcium in milk and other foods is very important. Calcium is a mineral needed by our bodies to ensure strong bones and teeth. A good supply of calcium is especially important during pregnancy (when your baby's bones and teeth are developing) and while breastfeeding.

Can't drink milk?

Some people strongly dislike milk and feel that it disagrees with their digestion. They may be allergic to milk or they may react badly to lactose, the sugar in milk.

In order to digest lactose, our bodies need an enzyme (special chemical) called lactase. Babies have plenty of lactase, but some adults have very little. These adults are unable to drink milk – but may find they can eat cheese and yoghurt because the lactose in these foods has been changed or removed. They may also be able to tolerate butter.

All of the nutrients in milk can be found in other foods, but it may be hard to get enough calcium if you dislike all dairy products. We suggest other sources of calcium in Chapter 2.

How much milk?

We need three servings of milk, or milk-based food, each day. A serving of milk is equivalent to:

- ❏ a full glass of milk (one-third of a pint or 200ml)
- ❏ a small carton of yoghurt
- ❏ a piece of hard cheese the size of a small matchbox
- ❏ half a small tub of cottage cheese (55g)
- ❏ half a small tub of fromage frais (100g)

What is so bad about fats and sugar?

The tiny section remaining on our plate is for fatty and sugary foods. Fats and sugar are found in many, many foods – not only in butter, cream and all types of sugar, but 'hidden' in lots of processed foods. Did you know, for example, that a large sausage contains the equivalent of 3 teaspoons of fat, and a can of soft drink 8 teaspoons of sugar?

We do need some fat in our diet. Fat is a source of vitamins A, D and E and essential fatty acids. But we don't need to deliberately choose fatty foods – because we get quite enough of both from other, more healthy foods.

The problem with fats

There are several different types of fat; some are more healthy than others. The three main types of fat are:

❏ saturated
❏ monounsaturated, and
❏ polyunsaturated.

The basic building blocks of fat are called fatty acids. Each type of fat is made up of different fatty acids.

Most adults in the UK eat too much fat – especially saturated fat. Too much saturated fat increases our risk of heart disease. All types of fat can contribute to an unhealthy weight gain. This is because fats are a very concentrated source of energy. They also tend to make foods taste good.

Saturated fats

Saturated fats are found mainly in foods that come directly, or indirectly, from animals – lard, butter, cream, fatty meat, hard cheese, and foods made using animal fats, like biscuits and ready-made pastry. Coconut oil, palm oil and ghee are also rich in saturated fats – as is chocolate. We should all eat a lot less saturated fat.

Meat and cheese, however, supply other valuable nutrients as well as containing saturated fat. The way around this dilemma is to try to choose lean cuts of meat (we only need a little, remember). It is also a good idea to trim away visible fat, and avoid using extra fat when cooking the meat. If you eat a lot of cheese, you may like to choose a low-fat variety. And, try a low-fat spread instead of butter. Semi-skimmed milk is just as nutritious as whole milk.

Mono and poly: the unsaturated fats

Monounsaturated fats are found in many foods, including vegetable oil, olive oil, soft margarines, meat, fish, avocado, eggs and peanuts. Check the 'nutritional information' label on packaged food to see what type of fat each food contains.

Monounsaturated and polyunsaturated fats are better for you than saturated fats. Polyunsaturated fats tend to be liquid at room temperature – in contrast to saturated fats which are usually hard (think of butter, lard, fat on meat and so on). Polyunsaturated fats are found in soya and sunflower cooking oils, sunflower margarine, oily fish, nuts and seeds.

Oily fish

Fish and shellfish are a valuable source of protein, vitamins and minerals as long as they're properly stored, handled and cooked. We should aim for at least two servings of fish a week, including one of oily fish. However oily fish contain more dioxins and dioxin-like chemicals than other foods so, although there are benefits from eating oily fish regularly, some scientists caution us not to eat more than two portions a week. Oily fish include mackerel, herring, sardines, pilchards, salmon or trout.

Mercury is a toxin that affects the nervous system and can build up in the bodies of predatory fish. So currently, the Food Standards Agency recommends that pregnant or breastfeeding women, women who intend to become pregnant, and children should avoid eating shark, swordfish, marlin and more than one fresh tuna steak or two tins of tuna (140g) a week.

Essential fatty acids

Polyunsaturated fats are important because they contain essential fatty acids. These special fatty acids are called 'essential' because they cannot be made in our bodies – we have to get them from our food. They are needed for normal brain development and the production of some of the hormones necessary for a healthy pregnancy. (Hormones are special chemicals working in our bodies.)

There are two essential fatty acids: linoleic acid and linolenic acid. Linoleic acid is found mainly in nuts, and in plant oils such as sunflower, soya or corn oil. Good sources of the other essential fatty acid – linolenic acid – are oily fish (tinned or fresh sardines, mackerel and salmon), eggs and lean meat.

It is important to take in a balance of the two fatty acids. Unless you are on a very low-fat diet, you are probably taking enough linoleic acid, but most of us would benefit from eating more oily fish and so increasing our intake of the second essential fatty acid, linolenic acid. Scientific research suggests that women who eat more oily fish tend to have longer pregnancies and bigger babies (see previous box on p19).

Trans fats

Finally, we need to mention a special group of fatty acids called 'trans fats'. You may notice on some spreads a label stating that 'This product contains virtually no trans fats'. This is because high intakes of trans fats have been linked with heart disease.

Trans fats are found in polyunsaturated fats that have been artificially processed in some way. For example, reheating vegetable oil changes the (healthy) fatty acids in that oil to (unhealthy) trans fats. A similar thing happens when liquid fats are hardened to use in factory-produced pastry and hard margarine. Butter, cream and cream cheese also contain some trans fats. The words 'hydrogenated vegetable oil (or fat)' on food labels means that the food probably contains trans fats.

We talk more about avoiding the unhealthy types of fats in Chapter 8.

What's wrong with sugar?

There are two main types of sugar:

❑ sugar added to foods
❑ basic sugars that are a natural part of nutritious foods like fruit, vegetables and milk.

The main problem with added sugar is that, although it gives us an energy boost, it contains no other nutrients at all. In fact, because our bodies need to work to digest sugar, nutrients from other foods are wasted. Too much added sugar actually drains nutrients from our bodies.

Eating sugary foods fills us up – so we can't eat other, healthier foods. They also contribute to tooth decay and to easy weight gain. Sugary foods don't satisfy us for long – so we soon feel hungry again. Finally, sugary foods – cakes, chocolates and sweets – tend to be expensive. So, bad food value all round!

The problem is that many of us really like the taste of sugar. Some women find that they want to eat more sugary foods at certain times of their menstrual cycle – or at different stages of pregnancy. It can be very hard saying 'no' to a tube of sweets or bar of chocolate at times like this. Try to think instead about the other type of sugar – the natural sugar found in fruit or in milk. Foods containing this kind of sugar are rich in many nutrients. When you crave a sugary snack, reach for things like kiwi fruit, bananas and cherries, dried fruit, a slice of fresh bread, a couple of digestive biscuits or some unsalted nuts.

We talk more about cutting down on sugar and sugary foods in Chapter 8.

Last, but not least – water!

We all need to drink plenty of water and other fluids. A good intake of liquid throughout the day helps with the smooth running of virtually every part of our body. When we drink enough water our digestion works better, our joints ache less and our skin is softer. Drinking plenty of water can relieve and help prevent many ailments – headaches, constipation, urine infections.

Drinking more while you are pregnant may seem odd,

because many women already find they need to go to the toilet more often, especially at night. But there is a reason for this. When you are pregnant, your body contains extra blood and other fluids, to meet the needs of your baby – and your kidneys need to work harder to cope with the additional demands. It is important that you drink plenty to meet your baby's needs, and to keep yourself in good health. Cutting back on what you drink to avoid getting up to go to the toilet at night can be harmful. Pregnant women are prone to urine infections and constipation and a good intake of fluid will help prevent both of these problems.

During pregnancy, try to drink 6–8 glasses of water, or other fluids, each day – not counting milk or alcohol. Some women find cold tap water very refreshing; others prefer bottled or fizzy water, unsweetened fruit juices or weak squash (avoid those with added sugar!). Many women enjoy coffee or tea, including the fruit and herbal types, or alcohol-free wines and beers. (More about tea, coffee and alcohol in Chapter 6.) The main thing is to find drinks that you enjoy.

Urine infection

Signs of a urine infection may include pain when passing urine, needing to go to the toilet often, or needing to go very urgently. Your urine may be dark in colour, cloudy or smelly. If you are worried that you may have a urine infection, start drinking plenty of water to wash out the germs, and contact your family doctor or midwife.

In this chapter we have described a basic plan for balanced eating: plenty of starchy carbohydrates, lots and lots of fruit and vegetables, small amounts of protein and milk foods, tiny quantities of fatty and sugary food – and plenty of water and other fluids. Enjoy your food!

Key points

❑ A balanced meal contains plenty of starchy carbo-hydrates, lots of vegetables and fruit, small amounts of protein and dairy produce, and tiny quantities of fatty and sugary foods.

❑ Try to eat five servings of fruit and vegetables each day (fresh, tinned, frozen or dried). Remember that over-cooking will reduce the vitamin content of these foods.

❑ Aim for two servings of animal protein, or two to three servings of vegetable protein, each day.

❑ Try to have three servings of milk, or milk-based foods (cheese, yoghurt, and so on) each day.

❑ Choose foods low in fat and sugar to allow for the occasional treat of sweets or crisps. Remember that unsaturated fats are healthier than saturated fats.

❑ Water is important! Try to drink 6–8 glasses of water, or other fluid, each day. (This does not include milk or alcohol!)

2

More about healthy eating

In this chapter, we talk in more detail about some of the vitamins, minerals and other nutrients mentioned in Chapter 1.

Eating the kind of balanced diet described in Chapter 1 will ensure that you take in plenty of most vitamins and minerals without worrying about any extra foods or supplements. There are a few exceptions to this – the most significant one being folic acid, one of the B group of vitamins. This is a very important vitamin for pregnant women – and for women planning a pregnancy.

There are a few other vitamins and minerals that certain groups of women may need to take special note of: for example, vitamin B_{12} if you eat a vegan diet, iron if you had very heavy periods before pregnancy, and vitamin D if you rarely go out of doors. Read on to find out more.

Folic acid: a very important vitamin for babies

Important: if you suffer from epilepsy, it is important to see your doctor before taking a folic acid supplement. Better still talk to him or her before you become pregnant.

Our bodies need folic acid (sometimes called folate) to make DNA. DNA carries the genetic information that controls the correct development and function of every single cell in our bodies. When you are pregnant, you need extra folic acid – especially in the first 12 weeks while your baby's body is being formed.

Insufficient folic acid at this time can contribute to problems with the neural tube of your developing baby. The neural tube develops in the very early weeks of pregnancy. It eventually forms your baby's brain and spinal cord (the long bundle of nerves inside our backbones that connects our brains with the rest of our bodies). You may have seen, or heard, the abbreviation NTD – this stands for neural tube defect. The most common type of neural tube defect is spina bifida. If you decide to have an ultrasound scan during your pregnancy, your baby's spine will be checked for signs of spina bifida.

Although NTDs are rare, the UK government advises all pregnant women to take folic acid supplements and eat more foods rich in folic acid. Extra folic acid is particularly important for women who have already had a baby with a neural tube problem.

Folic acid supplements

Folic acid supplements are available on prescription from your GP or midwife. NHS prescriptions are free to pregnant women. If you are not pregnant, you may have to pay for your prescription. In this case, it is cheaper to buy a folic acid supplement from a chemist or supermarket. Ask the pharmacist for advice.

Most folic acid supplements are small, white tablets. The recommended dose is 0.4mg each day. (This is sometimes written as 400µg, 400mcg or 400 microgrammes.) Much higher doses are given to women who have already had a baby with an NTD – ask your GP for guidance.

As well as taking a folic acid supplement, increase the amount of folic acid in your diet. This is good advice for all women – pregnant or not! Remember that folic acid, like most vitamins, is easily destroyed by cooking. It is therefore best to steam, microwave or stir-fry vegetables rich in folic acid – or cook in the minimum of water. Don't overcook!

Planning a pregnancy?

The government also advises that women planning to become pregnant should take folic acid supplements. This is because the neural tube develops during the first four weeks of pregnancy – when a woman may not realise she is pregnant. However, because many pregnancies are unplanned, this is not always possible. If you find yourself in this position, start taking a folic acid supplement as soon as possible, and increase the amount of folic acid in your diet. Remember that NTDs are relatively uncommon.

Foods rich in folic acid (best first)

❏ green leafy vegetables – brussels sprouts, spinach and broccoli
❏ other vegetables – green beans, potatoes, cauliflower, peas and cabbage
❏ tinned baked beans
❏ citrus fruits – oranges, orange juice and grapefruit
❏ fortified breakfast cereals (fortified means that extra nutrients have been added to the food – check the nutritional information chart on the packet)
❏ bread – especially fortified bread (check the label) and wholemeal bread
❏ yeast extract and beef extract
❏ milk

Vitamin B_{12}: another B group vitamin

There are many B group vitamins. Eating a balanced diet will give us plenty of all of them – except perhaps for folic acid and vitamin B_{12}.

Vitamin B_{12} (or 'cobalamin') is needed, like folic acid, for the production of new cells – especially new red blood cells. It also contributes to a healthy nervous system and is involved in the making of fatty acids. Vitamin B_{12} is therefore particularly important during pregnancy.

Vitamin B_{12} is found naturally only in foods that come from animals – meat, fish, eggs, milk and so on. It is also added to some breakfast cereals during their manufacture. It is very rare for women who eat animal foods to be deficient in vitamin B_{12}.

Women who do not eat meat will probably still get enough vitamin B_{12} from other animal foods, but women who do not eat any animal produce at all (a vegan diet) can become short of vitamin B_{12}. If you follow a vegan (or near vegan) diet, it is a good idea to eat plenty of fortified foods, and consider a B_{12} supplement. Ask your family doctor or a pharmacist to recommend a suitable supplement.

Foods rich in vitamin B$_{12}$ (best first)

- ❏ lamb's kidney
- ❏ other meat – beef, pork, lamb, sausages
- ❏ fish – such as cod, tinned sardines and pilchards
- ❏ eggs
- ❏ milk and hard cheese
- ❏ breakfast cereals – only fortified ones (check the nutritional information chart on the carton)
- ❏ soy 'meat' and soya milk are often fortified with vitamin B$_{12}$

Vitamin A: harmful if you have too much

We all need small amounts of vitamin A to keep our skin healthy. A balanced diet containing a range of fruit and vegetables, margarine and eggs will provide all the vitamin A we need. There is no need to take extra during pregnancy.

It may be harmful to your developing baby to have too much of the animal form of vitamin A (retinol). There are two ways in which this may happen: first, if you eat large amounts of liver, and second, if you take supplements of either vitamin A or fish oil.

Animal liver and liver products may contain high levels of the animal form of vitamin A. This is related to the type of food on which the animals have been fed. It is therefore best that you do not eat liver, or foods made from liver (such as paté) while you are pregnant. It is OK to eat these foods once you have had your baby.

Fish oil supplements (tablets, capsules or medicine) may also contain high levels of the wrong type of vitamin A. Fish oil contains essential fatty acids – but it is better to eat oily fish like mackerel, herrings, pilchards and salmon, rather than take a supplement (but see box on page 19).

If you feel you need to take a vitamin supplement, avoid ones that contain the 'retinol' form of vitamin A. Too much (more than 3,300 microgrammes, or mcg or µg) of this type of vitamin A may harm your developing baby. The 'carotene' form of vitamin A is safe – so check the label carefully and ask your pharmacist for advice.

Vitamin C: needed every day

Our bodies need a good supply of vitamin C to help fight infection and disease, to repair damage within our bodies, and to help heal wounds. Vitamin C also plays a role in preventing anaemia (lack of iron in the blood). Unlike other vitamins, vitamin C cannot be stored in our bodies – so we need to eat some foods rich in vitamin C each day.

Some women may need more vitamin C than others. If you smoke, or cannot avoid the smoke of other people's cigarettes, your body needs more vitamin C. Similarly, if you have been ill, or have had surgery, or have suffered an injury, your body will be using large amounts of vitamin C. In these circumstances, it is a good idea to increase your intake of foods rich in vitamin C.

Foods rich in vitamin C (best first)

❏ citrus fruits – oranges, grapefruits
❏ citrus fruit juices – fresh juice can be expensive; carton juice is just as good
❏ green vegetables – brussels sprouts, broccoli, cabbage
❏ other fruit and vegetables – kiwi fruit, black-currants, tomatoes, green peppers
❏ potatoes (yes, really! – especially if thinly peeled or scraped)

Tips for preserving vitamins

❏ Cook vegetables whole or cut into large pieces – this reduces the loss of vitamins during cooking. Try not to leave peeled vegetables soaking in water for a long time before cooking.

❏ When cooking vegetables on the hob, use only enough water to cover the vegetables. Bring the water to the boil, add the vegetables, cover the pan and boil briskly for a few minutes. Test the vegetables with a fork or knifepoint and stop cooking while the vegetables are still crisp. Leafy vegetables such as cabbage or spinach may only take 2–3 minutes to soften.

❏ Use the cooking water to make gravy or stock – to

save some of the vitamins that have seeped out into the water during cooking.

❏ Try steaming vegetables – it takes longer but is an excellent way of preserving both vitamins and taste (as is cooking in a microwave oven).

❏ Eat some vegetables raw: grated carrot and finely chopped white cabbage in coleslaw, chunks of sweet pepper, crispy stalks of celery – maximum vitamins and maximum taste!

❏ Eat most fruit raw – but do wash first in plenty of cold running water.

❏ If you wish to cook fruit on the hob, use only a small amount of water and cook gently, for as little time as possible. Redcurrants or ripe plums need only a moment's cooking – delicious on breakfast cereals or mixed into plain yoghurt.

❏ Try baking large apples or bananas in the oven, wrapped in foil with a sprinkling of dried fruit and served with a dollop of low-fat fromage frais.

❏ Vitamin C is easily destroyed by cooking. If you need to cook vitamin C foods, use only a small amount of water and cook for as little time as possible.

Antioxidants: nutrients fighting pollution

Antioxidants are a special group of nutrients that work to protect our bodies by blocking the action of 'free radicals'.

Free radicals are molecules (groups of particles) produced by our bodies. They are produced during many normal body processes – for example, the destruction of bacteria (germs) by our white blood cells, and the digestion of essential fatty acids. A certain level of free radicals is therefore normal.

The problem is that levels of free radicals within our bodies seem to be rising, as more and more are produced in response to pollutants such as cigarette smoke, exhaust fumes, and other toxic substances. If left unchecked, free radicals damage the cells of our bodies and weaken our defences against diseases such as heart disease and cancer.

The main antioxidants are:

❑   vitamins C and E
❑   two minerals called selenium and zinc
❑   beta carotene (the safe form of vitamin A).

Vitamin C is probably the most effective antioxidant. Most fruit and vegetables are good sources of vitamin C, especially citrus fruits, kiwi fruit, blackcurrants, peppers, tomatoes and green leafy vegetables. Vitamin E is found in vegetable oils, wholegrain bread and cereals, avocado pears and other green vegetables, eggs, butter and margarine.

We can get zinc from lean meat, cheese, milk, wholemeal bread and cereals. Cereals are also a good source of selenium, along with fish, pork, cheese, eggs and brazil nuts. Two other mineral antioxidants – copper and manganese – are found in wholegrain cereals, nuts, vegetables, meat and fish.

Beta carotene (and similar nutrients) are found in yellow and orange fruits such as mangoes, apricots, peaches and plums. Green leafy vegetables are rich in beta carotene, as are carrots, pumpkins and tomatoes. Cooked and processed tomatoes, in particular, are considered to be an excellent source of lycopene, another useful antioxidant.

Antioxidants are important for all of us, whether pregnant or not. A balanced diet, with plenty of fruit, vegetables and wholegrain bread and cereals will provide plenty of antioxidants.

Vitamin D: the sunlight vitamin

Vitamin D helps our bodies absorb and use a mineral called calcium. Calcium is needed for strong bones and teeth. A good intake of calcium is especially important during pregnancy when your baby's bones and teeth are developing.

Vitamin D is found in oily fish, such as sardines and mackerel, eggs, milk and other dairy products, and fortified foods such as margarine and breakfast cereals. Vitamin D is also made within our bodies, a process started by sunlight on our skins. People who spend some time out of doors each day, and who eat plenty of foods rich in vitamin D, usually have good stores of the vitamin.

The UK government recommends that pregnant (and breastfeeding) women should take a supplement of 10µg of vitamin D each day (sometimes written as 10mcg or 10 microgrammes). This is because some women in the UK may not build up adequate stores of vitamin D to meet the extra needs of pregnancy. You may like to talk to your GP about a vitamin D supplement if:

- you do not eat milk foods, and other animal foods such as fish and eggs
- you do not spend some time out of doors between 11am and 3pm each day (it doesn't matter if the sun isn't shining)
- you usually cover your arms, legs and head when out of doors
- you live in the north of England or in Scotland, where the winter days are short.

Calcium: a mineral for strong bones and teeth

Calcium and vitamin D are closely connected because we need vitamin D to help our bones and teeth make use of calcium. Dairy products are the best source of calcium.

One piece of research suggests that not having enough calcium may mean that some women are more likely to develop pre-eclampsia – but more proof is needed.

Foods rich in calcium (best first)

- ❏ milk, yoghurt and hard cheese (soft cheeses, like cottage cheese and cream cheese, also contain calcium – but less than hard cheeses such as parmesan, Cheddar and Double Gloucester)
- ❏ tinned fish – especially sardines and pilchards (including the soft bones!) and salmon
- ❏ soya milk and tofu (made from soya) often have calcium added (check the labels – the normal level for cow's milk is 120mg in 100ml)
- ❏ foods made using white flour (which is fortified with calcium) – white bread, pizza bases and pastry
- ❏ spinach and spring greens
- ❏ chick-peas, kidney beans and tinned baked beans
- ❏ sesame seeds and almonds
- ❏ oranges and dried figs

Zinc: the fertility mineral

Zinc plays an important part in fertility (getting pregnant) and healthy pregnancy. It is also needed for growth and healing, and for good immunity to infections and disease. Meat, milk foods and seafood are all good sources of zinc. Some experts are concerned that the absorption of zinc by our bodies can be reduced by an excessive amount of fibre in our diets, and by unnecessary iron and folic acid supplements. This is one reason why it is important to consult your GP, midwife or pharmacist before taking any nutritional supplements during pregnancy.

Foods rich in zinc (best first)

- ❏ meat – beef, lamb
- ❏ sardines – especially good for zinc!
- ❏ cashew nuts, lentils and chick-peas
- ❏ wholemeal bread
- ❏ other fish – smoked mackerel and prawns
- ❏ hard cheese, milk and eggs
- ❏ baked potatoes
- ❏ sunflower seeds and peanuts

Iron: for healthy blood

Iron is needed to make haemoglobin, a pigment that is found in our red blood cells. Haemoglobin carries oxygen around our bodies. If our red blood cells are not healthy, the transport of oxygen around our bodies may not be good enough. We may begin to feel tired, breathless, dizzy and miserable. These are some of the signs of anaemia.

Doctors and midwives used to give all pregnant women supplements of iron routinely. We now know that unnecessary iron supplements may interfere with the absorption of other minerals, such as zinc. They may also cause constipation. It is usually better to prevent anaemia by eating more iron-rich foods. Iron supplements are, however, necessary to treat anaemia; your doctor or midwife will advise you as to whether you need an iron supplement.

Foods rich in iron (best first)

❏ lean beef, lamb and kidney
❏ dark chicken or turkey meat
❏ fortified breakfast cereals
❏ sardines
❏ wholemeal bread
❏ red lentils, chick-peas, baked beans, kidney beans
❏ leafy vegetables – broccoli, peas, curly kale, spring greens, spring onions, spinach
❏ cashew nuts, sunflower seeds
❏ dried fruits – apricots, prunes and figs
❏ baked potatoes
❏ eggs

Tips on getting plenty of iron from your food

❏ Eat some food rich in vitamin C with every meal – fresh fruit or vegetables. This will help your body absorb iron, especially from non-meat iron foods. Vegetables such as peas, broccoli and spinach contain vitamin C as well as iron – provided they are not over-cooked. Spring onions are also full of vitamin C and iron – a convenient no-cook snack!

❏ Eat a variety of leafy green vegetables. (Spinach contains plenty of iron but this iron is not well absorbed by our bodies – so try other vegetables as well.)

❏ Eat meat or fish with non-meat iron foods. This will help you absorb as much iron as possible from the non-meat food – for example, minced beef eaten with leafy green vegetables.

❏ Drink tea and coffee between meals – rather than with your food. Both drinks contain chemicals that can reduce the amount of iron that your body can absorb from food. If you drink tea, have a cup an hour before your meal – or two hours afterwards.

❏ Certain foods reduce the amount of iron that our bodies can absorb from a meal. One example is rhubarb!

What about salt?

Most of us eat more salt than we need. Processed foods — such as ham, cheese, bread, baked beans and biscuits — all contain lots of salt. Savoury spreads (like yeast extract and beef extract), crisps, olives and salted nuts are obviously salty foods. In the long term, too much salt in your diet may contribute to high blood pressure and related health problems later in your life.

During pregnancy, however, the situation is more complicated. Restricting your salt intake at this time has not been shown to reduce the risk of high blood pressure during pregnancy. But this does not mean that you should add extra salt to your food. Use salt to flavour your food, as you would normally.

When you have had your baby, you can try reducing the amount of salt you use in cooking and on your food. This will help when your baby starts taking solid food, since babies should not have any salt at all added to their food.

There is no proof that cutting your salt intake during pregnancy will reduce swollen ankles. Similarly, there is no proof that leg cramps during pregnancy are caused by a lack of salt or of any other minerals.

Understanding food labels

What are calories?

A calorie (cal or kcal, for short) is a measure of how much energy a particular food gives us. Calories are sometimes called 'kilocalories'. They mean the same thing. A 'kilojoule' (kJ) is another measure of food energy. One calorie is equal to about 4 kilojoules.

What is the 'RDA'?

RDA stands for 'recommended daily amount'. The recommended daily amount of a certain nutrient is the amount that most of us need to keep healthy. RDAs vary from person to person. For example, children's nutritional needs are different from those of older people, and pregnant women's nutritional needs are different from those of men, or women who are not pregnant. Very active people need more energy than people who don't exercise much. The RDAs given on food labels usually refer to adult men.

Food labels usually list the RDAs of vitamins and minerals. The percentage figure given after each nutrient tells us how much of our RDA would be met by a portion of that particular food. For example, 'Folic acid 34mg (17%)' means that the food would give us 34mg of folic acid – or 17% of the daily requirement. This sounds very good – but remember that the RDA used is that of an adult man, rather than a pregnant woman whose need is much greater.

Next time you pick up an item of packaged food – a loaf of bread or a tin of baked beans, maybe – take a look at the panel of 'Nutritional Information' on the label. This information can be very useful when planning a balanced diet – especially when deciding whether or not to include a new food.

In Chapter 1 we used 'servings' to describe how much of each food group we need. We did not include weights because we feel that most women prefer not to spend their time weighing food and calculating the nutritional content of each item. Sometimes, however, it is useful to know just what a new food would contribute to your diet.

Imagine, for example, that you are trying to choose between two brands of breakfast cereal. The short list below suggests how much of each food group we need, in grams (usually written simply as 'g'). With these figures in mind, you can look at the amounts written on the Nutritional Information of the two cereals and see what proportion of that need would be met by an average portion of each one.

Each day during pregnancy the average woman needs:

❑ about 51g protein
❑ about 18g fibre
❑ as little sugar as possible – ideally no more than 50g
❑ as little saturated fat as possible – certainly no more than 23g
❑ no more than 53g of other fats
❑ about 15mg (milligrams) of iron
❑ about 2,000kcal of energy – or 8,100kJ (with an additional 200kcal during the last three months).

But things are not always as they appear! Sometimes interpreting food labels needs a bit of detective work.

The 'average serving' for each of these two foods is different because a cereal bowl can hold more toasted oat cereal than flakes. The values for the flakes includes nearly a quarter of a pint of milk. This makes it harder to compare the two cereals.

Both cereals contain relatively small amounts of protein – there's more protein in the milk than the cereals.

Toasted oat cereal with raisins
Ingredients: oat flakes, sugar, vegetable oil including hydrogenated vegetable oil, raisins, desiccated coconut, flaked almonds, sesame seeds, sunflower seeds, salt

	per 100g	per 50g serving (without milk)
energy	1,946kJ	973kJ
	463kcal	231kcal
protein	10.7g	5.4g
carbohydrate	57.9g	29.0g
(of which sugars)	(20g)	(10g)
fat	19.1g	9.6g
(of which saturates)	(5.8g)	(2.9g)
(polyunsaturates)	(2.7g)	(1.4g)
fibre	7.9g	4g
sodium	0.1g	0.1g

Manufacturers have to quote the nutrient content of 100g, but the figures for an 'average serving' are sometimes more helpful.

Although both cereals contain quite a lot of sugar, the toasted oat cereal contains less than half as much as the flakes.

A serving of the toasted oat cereal contains three times as much fibre as the flakes.

A bowl of flakes gives us much less energy than a bowl of toasted oat cereal. The toasted oat cereal contains more fibre and fats, so it will be digested more slowly and will keep hunger away longer.

Chocolate flake breakfast cereal
Ingredients: maize, sugar, milk chocolate, cocoa powder, salt, malt, vitamins

	per 100g	per 30g serving (with 125ml semi-skimmed milk)
energy	1,600kJ	380kJ
	380kcal	171kcal
protein	5g	5.6g
carbohydrate	84g	31.5g
(of which sugars)	(39g)	(17.9g)
(starch)	(45g)	(13.5g)
fat	2.5g	2.7g
(of which saturates)	(1.5g)	(1.7g)
fibre	2.5g	0.7g
sodium	0.9g	0.3g

The toasted oat cereal contains a lot more fat than the flakes. Some of these fats are polyunsaturates. These are the healthier types of fat. We are not told what proportion of the fats are trans fats.

There is just one thing the labels don't tell us – how a food tastes!

Key points

❏ Folic acid is very important, especially during early pregnancy. Take a 0.4mg supplement each day, and eat more foods rich in folic acid (leafy vegetables, tinned baked beans, fortified breakfast cereals).

❏ Women who eat a vegan, or near vegan, diet generally need a vitamin B_{12} supplement. Other women will get enough vitamin B_{12} from a balanced and varied diet.

❏ A balanced diet will provide all the vitamin A you need. Do not take a supplement.

❏ Try to eat some foods rich in vitamin C every day. A good intake of vitamin C is needed to fight infection and disease, and boost the absorption of iron from food. Remember that vitamin C is easily destroyed by cooking.

❏ Women who do not eat milk-based foods, or who do not spend much time out of doors may need a supplement of vitamin D.

❏ It is better to prevent anaemia by eating more iron-rich foods (meat, fortified breakfast cereals, beans, leafy vegetables) than to take an iron supplement.

3

Safety first

Pregnancy is a time to enjoy a rich variety of foods. It is also a time to take care of yourself and your growing baby by keeping in mind a few basic guidelines on food choice and preparation.

In this chapter we talk about the foods that may cause problems for you and your baby during pregnancy, and suggest ways in which you can avoid these problems.

'Why do I have to be so careful?'

'It's all so confusing. There seems to be endless lists of things I can't eat. When I was pregnant last time, I went to a family party. I put some home-made mayonnaise on my salad without thinking and spent the next six months worrying.'

'I feel like a child again with people saying "don't eat this, don't eat that". It's all rather patronising.'

Throughout pregnancy your baby is protected, floating in warm fluid contained within a bag of strong membranes, safe inside your uterus (womb). Her gateway to the world – to your body – is the placenta (afterbirth). Within the placenta, oxygen and nutrients pass from your blood to your baby's circulation, and carbon dioxide and other waste products are washed away.

The placenta is also a protective barrier. It filters out most bacteria, some drugs and other harmful substances. However, viruses (germs which are smaller than bacteria) and some bacteria can pass through.

Most of the germs with which we come into contact are harmless. There are, however, a few germs that may cause severe illness in babies. Examples include the virus that causes rubella (German measles), the listeria bacteria and the toxoplasmosis parasite.

The effect of these on the baby's development depends on how advanced the pregnancy is when her mother comes into contact with the germ. Your baby's immune system starts working during the fourth month of pregnancy and is then able to fight off many infections. (The immune system is an important part of our bodies' defence against infection and other illness.) In addition, your baby's body is fully formed by the fourth month of pregnancy. This means that she may not be so badly affected by an illness after this stage of pregnancy.

Changes during pregnancy

You may have noticed a warning message on recipes or menus advising that 'young children, elderly people, pregnant women and those suffering from immune-deficiency diseases' should avoid raw or lightly cooked eggs. This message appears because these people have a greater risk than other people of becoming very ill if they come into contact with salmonella bacteria (and other bacteria). This does not mean that while you are pregnant you are unwell or unduly delicate; it is simply a reflection of the normal changes happening to your immune system at this time.

Because of these changes, some bacteria are more dangerous to women when they are pregnant than at other times. Most forms of food poisoning do not directly harm babies, but their mothers may become very ill. Others, such as toxoplasmosis and listeria, can damage the baby, whilst causing only mild illness in the mother.

Most women keep as healthy as ever during pregnancy. A varied diet and regular exercise that you enjoy will help ward off coughs and colds and your immune system will return to normal soon after the birth of your baby.

'I'm still feeling a bit sick. I know I shouldn't eat certain things – but I feel I'm missing out on foods that I could really enjoy.'

'I'm not neurotic about it – if I make a mistake, I try to be realistic.'

What foods should I avoid?

It's OK to eat	Best to avoid	Why?
Hard cheeses such as Cheddar, Cheshire, Wensleydale, Edam, Gouda and parmesan. Soft, processed cheeses such as Philadelphia, DairyLea, mozzarella, cottage cheese, cream cheese, curd cheese. These are all safe, even if not marked as 'pasteurised'.	All soft, ripened cheeses such as Brie and Camembert. All blue-veined cheeses such as Stilton and Danish Blue. Other 'gourmet' cheese marked 'unpasteurised'. Some experts also recommend avoidance of feta cheese.	There is a small risk that these cheeses may contain the listeria bacteria, which can cause an illness called listeriosis.
Vegetable paté; meat pastes in jars; tinned paté; pasteurised, vacuum–packed paté; pasteurised paté in tubes – but not liver paté.	All fresh patés – especially liver paté. Avoid all liver and liver products, such as liver sausage and liver paté.	These foods may carry the listeria bacteria. In addition, liver and liver products are rich in the animal form of vitamin A and it is best to avoid high levels of vitamin A during pregnancy.
Cooked–chilled 'convenience' meals and ready-to-eat poultry which has been thoroughly reheated. (Preheat your oven, follow the manufacturer's instructions very carefully, and make sure that foods are piping hot right to the middle before eating.)	Unheated cooked–chilled meals. Poultry foods that have been pre-cooked and then chilled and which you cannot reheat safely before eating, such as roast chicken drumsticks and meat pies. Bought chicken and turkey sandwiches.	These foods may contain the listeria bacteria.

Packaged pies and pasties, date-stamped and bought from a busy, reputable shop.	Cold foods sold loose from delicatessen counters.	These foods may contain the listeria bacteria and other germs which may cause food poisoning.
Salads made from fresh, well-washed ingredients and dressed salads prepared immediately before eating.	Ready-prepared and packaged salads straight from the bag and ready-made dressed salads (such as potato salad or coleslaw).	These may carry the listeria bacteria. Dirty salad ingredients may carry the toxoplasmosis parasite.
Eggs cooked until both the yolk and the white are solid. Commercially produced mayonnaise in jars and other products made using pasteurised eggs. Home-made desserts, icing and so on made using pasteurised egg.	Raw or undercooked eggs in any form; sorbet, mousse, meringue, home-made mayonnaise.	There is a small risk that eggs and egg products may carry the salmonella bacteria which can cause severe food poisoning.
Packaged ice cream and ice lollies kept in a freezer.	Soft, whipped ice cream sold from vans or kiosks.	There is a small risk that this may contain salmonella and other bacteria.
Well-cooked poultry and meat, cooked until no meat remains pink and the juices run clear.	Raw, 'rare' or undercooked poultry and meat of any kind.	Undercooked meat may contain the salmonella bacteria. It may also carry the toxoplasmosis parasite.

Continued

It's OK to eat	Best to avoid	Why?
Well-washed raw vegetable and salad items.	Unwashed vegetables. Even packaged, supermarket fruit and vegetables should be thoroughly washed under running water.	Unwashed vegetables and salad items may be contaminated with the toxoplasmosis parasite and germs which may cause food poisoning.
Cooked shellfish as part of a hot, well-cooked meal.	Raw shellfish such as oysters, mussels, cold prawns, crab.	These foods may contain bacteria that can cause severe food poisoning.
Pasteurised, sterilised or ultra-heat-treated (UHT) milk. Unpasteurised milk boiled for two minutes before use in puddings or drinks is also considered safe.	Untreated, 'green top' milk from cows, sheep or goats.	Untreated milk may be a source of brucellosis and other bacteria, which can cause food poisoning. It may also carry the listeria bacteria. Goat's milk may contain the toxoplasmosis parasite.

Listeriosis

Listeriosis is the illness caused by the listeria bacteria. Listeriosis can feel a bit like a mild bout of 'flu with aches and pains, a raised temperature and maybe a sore throat. Some people may not even be aware that they are ill; this is called a 'silent infection'. Listeriosis is usually only a problem if the infection passes from a pregnant woman to her unborn baby.

If a woman catches listeriosis early in pregnancy she may have a miscarriage. Later in pregnancy, listeriosis may cause premature labour or stillbirth. If a woman catches listeriosis during the last few weeks of pregnancy, her baby may be very ill when she is born.

The listeria bacteria can be found in the soil, on vegetation, and in some foods. It cannot be caught by touching, or breathing it in – only by eating it in contaminated food. Listeria is an unusual germ in that it can grow slowly at low temperatures, even inside a fridge. The good news is that listeria bacteria are easily killed by adequate cooking.

Blue-veined cheeses carry a particular risk of listeriosis. This is because the ripening process (which creates the blue veins) encourages the growth of listeria bacteria. While you are pregnant (and, if possible, when you are planning to become pregnant), it is best to avoid all blue-veined cheeses, white-skinned, ripened cheeses and patés.

Using convenience foods

Other foods, such as convenience meals and pre-cooked poultry, may be contaminated with listeria during preparation. The germs may then multiply during storage, even in a supermarket chill cabinet or domestic fridge.

Use convenience foods with care:

❏ eat foods before their 'use by' or 'eat by' date, before any germs they may contain can multiply to dangerous levels

❏ follow the manufacturer's instructions carefully, allowing time for your oven to heat to the correct temperature

❏ if using a microwave oven, check that you are following the instructions appropriate to the power of your oven

❏ before eating the food, slice or stir it to be sure that the middle is piping hot.

Sometimes you may wish to reheat food that is not packaged and carries no specific instructions – maybe a chicken pie bought from a local baker. The middle of the pie needs to be at a temperature of 70°C for at least two minutes to kill the listeria bacteria. To reach this kind of 'core' temperature, food should be reheated at 180°C (350°F or gas mark 4) for about 20 minutes. At the end of this time, cut through the pastry to make sure that the filling is steaming and piping hot. If it is not, cover the food with foil and return it to the oven for another 5–10 minutes.

Remember that listeriosis is a rare illness, affecting about one pregnancy in every 30,000. If you do your best to avoid the foods that may carry the bacteria, you are very, very unlikely to catch listeriosis. Even if you eat one of the foods by mistake, your risk is still extremely small.

If, at any time during pregnancy, you are worried that you may have been in contact with the listeria bacteria, contact your GP quickly. Listeriosis can be diagnosed by blood or urine test and antibiotic treatment may be helpful.

Salmonella

There are many germs that can cause food poisoning. The salmonella bacterium is probably one of the most common. Salmonella food poisoning can be very unpleasant. After eating food contaminated with salmonella, people may become extremely unwell, with severe vomiting, diarrhoea, a high temperature and dehydration. Treatment generally involves antibiotics and replacement of fluid lost by the body. Hospital treatment is occasionally needed. When you are pregnant you are more likely than at other times to be badly affected by salmonella bacteria and other germs responsible for food poisoning.

Another cause of food poisoning is the campylobacter bacterium. These bacteria can cause diarrhoea and stomach cramps. As with salmonella, your baby will not be directly harmed, but it is sensible to try to avoid the bacteria for your own health and wellbeing.

Salmonella and eggs

It has been estimated that about one egg in every 450 is contaminated by salmonella bacteria. Thorough cooking kills the bacteria. Eggs that have been cooked until both the white and the yolk are solid are safe.

Use eggs with care:

❑ a medium–sized egg (size 2) should be boiled for at least seven minutes

❑ poach eggs until the white of the egg is completely solid and opaque, and the yolk is set firm (a medium-sized egg will take about five minutes)

❑ fry eggs on both sides

❑ use pasteurised egg products for recipes involving the use of raw or only lightly cooked egg, such as royal icing, mayonnaise or meringue (pasteurised egg products can be found in larger supermarkets).

Eggs are not the only source of salmonella germs. The bacteria can be found in many raw foods that have been handled with dirty hands or utensils. Later in this chapter we outline the main ways in which we can all guard ourselves, and our families, against the risk of food poisoning. These guidelines are not just for pregnancy; many other people are at risk of severe food poisoning. And, of course, nobody – young or old, pregnant or not – wants to fall ill when it can be prevented.

Toxoplasmosis

Toxoplasmosis is an illness caused by a tiny parasite called *Toxoplasma gondii*. The parasite may be found in raw meat (especially lamb), soil, dirty vegetables and cat faeces. It may also be found in goat's milk. The parasite can only be caught by eating contaminated food or by licking dirty hands. Following the general guidelines in the section on food safety later in this chapter will help reduce your risk of coming into contact with toxoplasmosis.

Toxoplasmosis generally causes a mild, 'flu-like illness but, like listeriosis, you may not even feel particularly unwell. Many people catch toxoplasmosis, make a full recovery and are then immune to the illness. About one-third of young adults in this country are immune to toxoplasmosis, so there is a good chance that you are already safe from the infection. Some antenatal clinics offer pregnant women a blood test to check their immunity to toxoplasmosis.

Like listeriosis, toxoplasmosis is really only a problem to babies who are still developing inside their mothers' wombs. If a woman becomes infected with toxoplasmosis, the parasite can cross the placenta and infect her baby. The damage caused to the baby would depend on the stage of the pregnancy. The most dangerous time is the first half of pregnancy. Toxoplasmosis can cause many problems, including harm to the baby's developing brain and eyes.

Toxoplasmosis and cats

The toxoplasmosis parasite sometimes lives and multiplies inside infected cats and is passed out in their faeces. This is why it is sensible for pregnant women (and women planning a pregnancy) to wear gloves while gardening or handling soil. Even if you do not own a cat, neighbouring cats may have visited your garden and used it as a toilet. When you have finished gardening, store your gloves well away from where you prepare food, and wash your bare hands thoroughly with soap and warm water.

Handle cat dirt and litter with care:

❏ if possible, ask somebody else to empty your cat's litter tray

❏ wear rubber gloves and use a scoop or small trowel when tidying or emptying your cat's litter tray

❏ wrap the dirty litter in several sheets of newspaper and place the parcel directly in your dustbin

❏ wash your gloved hands before removing your gloves

❏ store your gloves well away from where you prepare food

❏ wash your bare hands thoroughly with soap and warm water, in case any small grains of litter have trickled down inside the gloves.

Although toxoplasmosis can have very nasty effects, it is rare for unborn babies to be harmed. It has been estimated that one baby in every 50,000 births will be affected by toxoplasmosis.

> If you are worried that you may have caught toxoplasmosis, arrange to see your GP urgently. The infection can be diagnosed with a blood test and, if necessary, drugs will be given to reduce the risk of the parasite passing across to your baby.

Vitamin A

Vitamin A is a valuable and necessary part of our diet. We get all the vitamin A we need from a balanced diet; we do not need supplements.

Too much of the animal form of vitamin A during pregnancy can cause developmental problems in unborn babies. For this reason, it is not a good idea to take supplements of vitamin A (including capsules or tablets of fish liver oils) while you are pregnant. More than 3,300µg of vitamin A daily can be dangerous. (This dose is sometimes written as 3.3mg, 3,300mcg or 3,300 microgrammes.)

Experts also recommend that pregnant women (and women planning to become pregnant) do not eat liver and liver products during pregnancy. This is because liver can contain very high levels of retinol vitamin A. Similar levels may also be found in liver products such as liver paté or liver sausage.

It is safe to eat liver when you are not pregnant. Liver is an excellent source of iron and is often recommended to women who may be anaemic. Other good sources of iron include red meat, fortified breakfast cereals and bread and green vegetables.

How to keep food safe

Remember the four basics!

- ❑ Keep germs out of food. Clean food, clean hands, clean kitchen.
- ❑ Stop germs multiplying in food. Cool quickly, store chilled.
- ❑ Destroy any germs in food by adequate cooking.
- ❑ Eat food soon once cooked.

Keep germs out of food

Remember that germs need to get onto food in the first place, and that food prepared in a clean way is unlikely to be contaminated with harmful bacteria.

Choose food carefully

Buy food that appears fresh and undamaged. Make sure that packaging is intact. Take note of manufacturers' 'use by' or 'eat by' dates and eat food before these are reached. Food eaten after these dates may be starting to go bad. The first signs are usually a change in taste and appearance: yoghurts taste fizzy, milk smells sour, lettuce becomes limp, and so on. The food will soon become less nutritious as levels of nutrients such as vitamin C decrease.

Store food carefully

Wash raw vegetables, or wrap them up well. Store them away from other foods. Soil clinging to raw vegetables may contain toxoplasmosis or other germs. Wash all fruit and vegetables before use – even clean, pre-packed supermarket produce may carry germs.

Always, always wash your hands before preparing food

Wash thoroughly, using any kind of soap and plenty of warm water. Take care to wash between fingers and around thumbs. Even if our hands are not visibly dirty, they may carry dangerous germs. Use a clean hand towel each day.

Remember that animals and kitchens do not mix

Keep household pets off tables and work surfaces. Prepare and serve animal food well away from where you prepare your own food. Use separate utensils for your pets, and wash their dishes and spoons separately from your own. Teach children from an early age to enjoy stroking their pets – but teach them also, by your words and example, to wash their hands afterwards.

Cats, dogs and other household pets bring enjoyment to many families and there is no doubt that children benefit from the presence of a safe family pet. But, however much we love our pets, we need to remember that they can carry unpleasant germs.

Keep work surfaces, dishcloths and other equipment scrupulously clean

Wipe tables, work surfaces and chopping boards with hot, soapy water before and after use. Germs on these surfaces will attach to the food you are preparing and traces of food left when you have finished work will attract flies and pets – and their germs.

Dishcloths should be changed at least every day, and machine- or hand-washed at a high temperature. You may prefer to use kitchen paper or disposable cloths such as 'J-Cloths'.

Use a clean tea towel and hand towel every day, and launder dirty ones at a high temperature.

You may have seen advertisements for antibacterial sprays and washing-up liquids – even chopping boards and towels. We are not sure how effective these are when used at home. If you decide to use these items, do remember that they cannot replace the hygiene measures outlined above.

Stop germs multiplying in food

Even if germs do get into food, most will not grow to dangerous levels if the food is kept well chilled, in an efficient refrigerator, until the very last moment before cooking.

Keep cold foods cold and make sure that your fridge is cold enough. Carry chilled or frozen foods home in an insulated bag or box. These can be bought in most supermarkets. If chilled food is allowed to warm up too much during the journey home, bacteria may begin to grow within the food. The temperature inside your fridge should be between 0°C and 4°C. Many supermarkets and hardware shops sell reasonably priced fridge thermometers – or you may be able to get one free from your local environmental health department.

Remember that listeria bacteria are unusual in that they can grow at low temperatures; this is why thorough reheating of chilled, pre-cooked food and ready-to-eat poultry is very, very important.

Cool quickly any foods that have been cooked but are to be used later

Cover cooked food and leave in a cool, draughty area for no longer than two hours. Divide large quantities of food into smaller containers to speed up cooling. Germs grow best when food is warm. Even slightly contaminated foods left for a long time at room temperature (especially in warm weather) will rapidly become dangerously full of bacteria.

Put the cooled food into the coldest part of your fridge (generally the lower shelves) until thoroughly chilled.

Be particularly careful with the storage of raw meat

Store raw meat at the bottom of your fridge or in a deep, covered dish. Make sure that the juice from raw meat cannot drip onto other food. Germs from raw meat may pass to cooked foods or fresh produce such as fruit, vegetables and dairy items.

Keep a separate chopping board on which to prepare raw meat. Use a permanent marker pen to write 'Raw meat only' on the underside of this board, or buy a different coloured board.

Do not put cooked foods down where raw foods have previously stood, without thoroughly cleaning the surface. When marinating raw meat, make sure the dish is covered and kept refrigerated. Wash hands, knives and other utensils carefully after preparing raw meat.

Take care with eggshells

Store eggs away from other foods, and wash your hands after handling the shells. Wipe shells just before you crack them. Cooking will kill any germs inside but the outside of the shells may also carry harmful bacteria.

Destroy any germs in food

Remember that adequate cooking will kill any bacteria lurking in raw meat, poultry and eggs.

Cook meat and poultry carefully

Follow cooking instructions carefully, but remember that some ovens are not so good as others are and some cuts of meat are harder to cook than others. When you feel that the meat has finished cooking, test it by sticking a fork or skewer into the thickest part of the meat. The meat is well cooked if the juices that trickle out are clear in colour. You will be able to enjoy raw or lightly cooked meat again as soon as your baby is born; while pregnant, it is best to cook meat thoroughly until you can see no pink meat or blood.

Be particularly careful with barbecued or grilled food; the outside of burgers, sausages and other food may appear cooked while the inside is still pink or red.

A large chicken or turkey may also cause problems; germs may survive in the middle even after long periods of slow cooking. Choose smaller poultry and calculate cooking time according to total weight, including any stuffing.

Eat food soon once cooked

Eat food as soon as it is ready. Food left waiting before being eaten may become contaminated with germs – from utensils, passing flies or fingers. Germs that have not been killed by cooking may start to grow. The longer that warm food is left, the greater the number of bacteria within it.

Try to avoid reheating food for a second time. Toxic substances may start to accumulate if warm food is left standing for a long time before being either eaten or chilled. The second reheating may not kill these poisons. The more often that food is heated and left warm, the greater the risk of contamination with germs. Also, food rapidly becomes less nutritious each time it is reheated.

Don't freeze food for a second time (unless it has been cooked in between). Once food is thawed, there is a chance that germs may start to grow within it. When the food is refrozen, the germs will also be frozen but will not be destroyed. Later cooking may not kill these germs.

It's not always easy

In our own kitchens we can make sure that food is pre-pared safely. Sometimes, though, things are out of our control. It can be hard to insist that things are done in a certain way if we share a kitchen with other people, whether family or strangers. And preparing and storing food in a safe way can also be extremely difficult without running water or a fridge.

In these situations it may help to shop 'little and often' to reduce the need for food storage. Try to keep meals simple to cut down on preparation. Remember that hand washing is probably the single most helpful thing you can do to keep food safe.

Sometimes using packaged and convenience foods may seem to be the only solution. These foods can certainly be very useful – but they can also be costly to buy. And, of course, we cannot control the way in which convenience foods are prepared by manufacturers; newspaper and TV reports of problems with commercial food production have alarmed us all. We can only trust that packaged foods produced by reputable manufacturers are prepared under hygienic conditions.

Remember the basics of food safety, keep meals simple, and enjoy your food.

Key points

❑ Wash hands well after gardening, handling animals, and dealing with cat litter. Wear gloves when possible.

❑ Wash hands before preparing food, and keep work surfaces, kitchen cloths and utensils clean.

❑ Choose food carefully, taking note of 'use by' and 'eat by' dates. Avoid soft, ripened cheeses, fresh paté, liver products, pre-cooked poultry that you cannot reheat, foods containing raw or lightly cooked eggs, soft ice cream and unpasteurised milk.

❑ Store food with care, keeping raw foods (including eggs) away from cooked foods. Wash fruit and vegetables well before use. Wipe eggshells before cracking open. Keep cold foods well chilled. Make sure your refrigerator works well.

❑ Cook meat and poultry thoroughly, and make sure that food is cooked right through. Follow carefully the reheating instructions on cooked-chilled foods, and check that food is piping hot to the middle. Cook eggs until both the white and the yolk are solid. Eat food soon after cooking, or cool quickly and store chilled for later use.

4

'But I feel so awful'

During the first three months of pregnancy your baby develops from a microscopic dot to a tiny, but fully formed, baby. Four weeks after conception her heart is beating, and a month later she begins to move!

However, many women find these early months of pregnancy very difficult. Some of the normal changes of pregnancy can spoil your enjoyment of food and make eating a balanced diet difficult. We suggest some things that you can try that may help.

Pregnancy sickness

'I was sick every hour. I felt utterly miserable – I couldn't even remember why I wanted to be pregnant in the first place.'

'Just once or twice, I felt a bit queasy – that was all!'

About 80% of women feel sick in the first three months of pregnancy. Some feel sick just in the morning, others in the evening – many feel sick off and on throughout the day. Some women vomit. Many women are sick just once or twice a week – others vomit several times a day. Just a few women become so ill that they need treatment in hospital.

Pregnancy sickness usually starts at 4–6 weeks of pregnancy. It tends to be at its worse at around 9–10 weeks, before getting a lot better by 12–16 weeks. A few women continue to feel ill off and on throughout their pregnancy, but most soon start to enjoy their food again.

Many women also notice changes in their senses of taste and smell. You may find that you suddenly dislike the taste of foods that you previously enjoyed – or you may notice an odd, maybe metallic, taste in your mouth. Other women find their sense of smell gets stronger and they dislike the smell of things like cooking, cigarette smoke or exhaust fumes.

Most women feel very tired during the first three months of pregnancy. You may find yourself nodding off at work or on a bus. You may sit down for a meal or to watch television and promptly fall asleep. Many women find this feeling of tiredness very alarming, and wonder how on earth they are going to manage for the nine months of pregnancy. But things do get better! Most women find that by their fourth or fifth month of pregnancy, they feel once again full of life and strength.

Why?

What causes pregnancy sickness? Nobody knows for sure, but there are several theories.

Your pregnancy is controlled by many different hormones. One of these hormones is called human chorionic gonadotrophin (hCG for short). Experts feel that this hormone may be partially responsible for pregnancy sickness. Levels of hCG rise rapidly during the first 6 weeks of pregnancy, reach a maximum at 8–10 weeks, and begin to fall at 11–13 weeks (when other hormones take over control). You may notice that your sickness follows a similar sort of pattern.

Rising levels of another hormone – progesterone – are thought to contribute to the feeling of tiredness. This hormone increases throughout pregnancy, but after three months or so it seems that your body becomes used to a high level of progesterone and you begin to feel less tired.

Feeling tired is closely connected to feeling sick. When we feel sick it is hard to eat, so the level of sugar in our blood falls, and we become tired and weak. Similarly, when we are tired (pregnant or not) – we often feel slightly sick. It can become a vicious circle. Giving in to the feeling of tiredness and resting often eases nausea.

Pregnancy sickness may also be caused, in part, by changes in your digestive system. Once again, progesterone is to blame. Progesterone causes some of the muscles in your body to become looser and softer during pregnancy. This is good because it allows your uterus to stretch to hold your growing baby. Another effect is to slow down the action of your gut, so food moves along more slowly and you feel fuller for longer. This may contribute to pregnancy sickness. On the other hand, the relatively slow movement of food through your system means that more nutrients can be absorbed and used by your body.

'What about my baby?'

The main thing to remember is that normal pregnancy sickness will not harm your baby. Even if you are eating very little, drinking only water, and vomiting several times a day, your baby will continue to develop and grow, using nutrients from the stores within your body.

Sickness seems to be a natural part of early pregnancy. Some experts feel that sickness is actually a sign that your pregnancy hormones are working well. It may be that women who feel sick are less likely to miscarry.

Pregnancy sickness and changes to your senses of taste and smell may even help protect your baby from things that may be harmful. Many women find that early in pregnancy they suddenly dislike alcohol and cigarettes. Both can be harmful to your growing baby.

Things that may help pregnancy sickness

Don't suffer in silence! Tell your midwife or doctor how you are feeling. Talk things over with your mother, sisters or friends. They will probably have many good, safe ideas to help you through this difficult part of your pregnancy (but do check with your midwife, doctor or pharmacist before taking any medicines or special foods).

Different things work for different women. Here are our suggestions.

Little and often

'I had to eat something every hour or so – otherwise I felt sick – so I went mad on bananas.'

'I kept a big packet of crisps in my desk – and I just kept eating them every 10 minutes – all day! It was the only thing that stopped me being sick.'

'Weetabix and milk – that's what kept me going.'

Although nobody knows for sure what causes pregnancy sickness, we do know that it is made worse by low levels of sugar in your blood. You feel sick, so you don't eat – and the sickness gets worse. This may be why pregnancy sickness is often worse in the morning – after not eating overnight. Alternatively, women who are unable to eat much during the day find they feel most nauseated in the evenings.

Many women find that it helps to eat little and often. Eat whatever your appetite suggests – even if it seems to be an unhealthy food, like crisps or sweets. Now is not the time to worry about putting on too much weight. Although your baby is still very tiny, many changes are already happening within your body. These changes all take energy. Pregnancy sickness may well be nature's way of telling you that you need to eat more – not less – to meet your body's needs.

Eat just small amounts so that your stomach does not become over-full, and eat often so that your blood sugar stays high. If you feel sick when you do not eat frequently, your body is telling you that you need more food. Trust it!

Later, when you feel better, you may find that you can substitute healthier snacks (lower in fat and sugar). Later still, when the sickness has passed, you can concentrate again on eating a balanced diet. But, for now, don't worry. Eat what you can, drink as much as you can – and take it one day at a time. It will get better.

Some women feel that they cannot bear to actually cook food, for themselves or for others. Is there anybody who can help you with cooking? Would it help to use more convenience foods for a few weeks? Alternatively, reassure yourself that appropriate raw foods are generally more nutritious than cooked ones.

How to tell when pregnancy sickness may be harmful

Contact your midwife or GP urgently if:

❏ you feel so sick that you cannot drink even water
❏ you are passing only small amounts of dark-coloured urine
❏ you have a fever

Nutritious snacks and quick, no-cook meals – for pregnancy and afterwards

- [ ] celery, carrots or pitta bread dipped in hummus
- [ ] chopped green or red peppers and tinned sweetcorn with tinned chick-peas
- [ ] grated carrot, raisins, peanuts, sunflower seeds
- [ ] celery, apple and pecans or walnuts on a bed of lettuce
- [ ] avocado pear – can be expensive, but high in energy and monounsaturated fats
- [ ] fresh fruit salad – keep a bowl ready in the fridge
- [ ] cold cooked pasta mixed with peas, tomatoes, cucumber and tuna, ham or chicken
- [ ] breadsticks, crackers, rice cakes
- [ ] breakfast cereal (any time!), preferably a low-sugar type served with skimmed or semi-skimmed milk
- [ ] wholemeal toast with yeast extract (Marmite)
- [ ] wholemeal bread with mashed banana
- [ ] wholemeal scones, muffins, crumpets – preferably with a low-fat spread
- [ ] natural or fruit yoghurt, fromage frais
- [ ] natural yoghurt and milk mixed together (maybe with a pinch of salt or sugar) – this is lassi, a refreshing Indian drink
- [ ] cheese cubes with apple, pineapple, chopped sweet pepper, cherry tomatoes

- ❏ cottage cheese – try adding your own chopped spring onions or fruit
- ❏ tinned fish – sardines, mackerel, salmon and so on
- ❏ tinned baked beans – packed with nutrients and fibre, hot or cold!
- ❏ sandwiches of all kinds – try to mix protein with fruit or vegetables: peanut butter and apple, tuna and tomato, turkey and beetroot.

Rest – as much as you can

'I felt so tired that sometimes I even had to stop when I was driving, pull over and have a 10-minute nap. I was in danger of falling asleep at the wheel.'

'I spent the first month or so sleeping, eating and being sick.'

It can be difficult finding the time to rest during the day – especially if you have not yet told family and work colleagues about your pregnancy. But even a short rest with your feet up and your eyes closed can make a dramatic difference to how you feel.

You may find it helpful to pinpoint the time in the day when you feel most unwell, and focus on arranging one good rest period around that time. If you feel worse in the morning, could you arrange to start work later, for a few weeks? If you feel ill later in the day, could you take a longer lunch-break and make up the work time in the evening? If things are really bad, could you take a few days' holiday? If you have a toddler at home, is there a regular TV programme that always holds her attention, giving you the chance to rest in an easy chair?

If you simply cannot rest during the day, try to go to bed early. Again, we know this can be difficult if older children need your attention, or your partner does not come home until late. Could you prepare food earlier in the day for other family members and leave it ready for them? What about the occasional take-away meal?

If you can't manage to rest during the day, or go to bed early, your baby will not be harmed – but if you can take it a little easier, you will probably feel a lot better, and other members of your family may also feel the benefits. Any arrangements you need to make will probably be for only a few weeks. The tiredness and the sickness will soon pass.

Ginger for pregnancy sickness

Research suggests that ginger, in various forms, may help ease pregnancy sickness. The evidence is not strong – but it is a safe and easy thing to try:

❑ drink ginger beer or ginger ale – both non-alcoholic and full of sugar (so good for energy levels, too)

❑ make ginger tea by putting a little grated ginger root (from larger grocers and most supermarkets) in a teapot, adding boiling water, and leaving to brew for 10–15 minutes. Add camomile or lemongrass tea to complement the flavour, or a few drops of lemon juice and some honey – and enjoy hot or cold

❑ use fresh ginger root in stir-fries and sauces for fish, chicken or pasta

❑ use dried ginger (sold in jars in the herbs and spices section of most grocers and supermarkets) in home-made biscuits and cakes

❑ buy ginger biscuits, gingerbread or parkin and look out for ginger marmalade or rhubarb and ginger jam.

❑ try crystallised ginger (chunks of preserved ginger, sold either in packets or in jars of syrup). Look for this in sweet shops or the 'home baking' section of supermarkets. It can be expensive – but think of it as a medicine!

Other ideas for coping with sickness

'I found sea-sickness bands really helpful during my first pregnancy – but they didn't seem to help at all the next time.'

'A friend of mine has had acupuncture – she said it was wonderful – the sickness just stopped. But it does seem a bit expensive.'

There is research evidence that supplements of vitamin B_6 (pyridoxine) relieve pregnancy sickness. If you are vomiting a lot, your levels of vitamin B_6 may get low. Sometimes vitamin B_6 is given with a mineral called magnesium. Some women find zinc helpful. Speak with your midwife or GP before taking any supplements.

When you can eat, it may be a good idea to concentrate on foods rich in zinc and the B group of vitamins. We list foods rich in zinc in Chapter 2. Foods rich in vitamin B_6 include:

❑ fortified breakfast cereals, wheatgerm
❑ baked potatoes, bananas, lentils, sunflower seeds
❑ mackerel, tuna, salmon, turkey, chicken.

Some women find that 'acupressure bands' work well. These are sold in larger chemists. Many people buy them to help relieve travel sickness, as well as pregnancy sickness. One brand name is 'Sea Bands'. They appear to work by putting continuous, gentle pressure on a certain acupressure point on the inside of your wrist. Pressure on this point relieves the nausea felt by people receiving strong drugs for the treatment of cancer.

It is important that you follow the fitting instructions very carefully. Acupressure bands are quite expensive – but should last through several pregnancies. If using them relieves your sickness, you may feel it money well spent! Acupressure bands do not work for everybody.

Other alternative therapies, such as acupuncture, homoeopathy, herbal medicine and reflexology, can also be helpful. It is important, though, that you discuss your needs with a qualified practitioner. Look in your local *Yellow Pages* phone book under 'Alternative Medicine'. Your midwife may also be able to advise you. Alternative medicine consultations and treatments can be very expensive so ask about costs before booking your first appointment. Always tell anybody advising you about your health that you are pregnant – or planning a pregnancy.

Choosing a take-away meal

Healthier choices include:

- ❏ baked potatoes
- ❏ Chinese or Thai-style stews and rice
- ❏ Indian meals – vegetable and meat dishes with plenty of rice or breads
- ❏ pitta bread with kebabs and plenty of salad.

Occasional treats only!

- ❏ fried prawn balls or crackers
- ❏ meat curries with visible fat
- ❏ individual meat pies, cornish pasties, samosas
- ❏ burgers, battered chicken pieces, sausages
- ❏ fish and chips (thick chips best!)

Heartburn

'It was miserable. I didn't know heartburn could be so bad! I must have got through thousands of antacid tablets.'

'I worked out that the days I had banana sandwiches I had worse heartburn. So I switched to Marmite toast, or yoghurt with raisins, and that seemed to help.'

Heartburn is an unpleasant, burning sensation in the oesophagus (gullet or food tube). It may be felt at intervals throughout the day, and is often worse after meals and at night. About half of all pregnant women have heartburn, generally in the last three months of pregnancy, although it can happen in early pregnancy too.

Heartburn is caused by small amounts of acid escaping into the gullet through the top opening of the stomach. (Gastric acids are strong chemicals in our stomachs which contribute to the digestion of our food.) Normally, the top opening of our stomach is firmly closed, except when food is passing down through it. However, during pregnancy, the hormone progesterone loosens the muscle enclosing this opening, so the gastric acids can leak out. This can happen when your stomach is over-full – maybe after a large meal. The pressure of your growing baby pushing against your stomach from below also contributes to heartburn. Many women find that heartburn gets worse when they bend over or lie down.

The pressure on your stomach is immediately relieved when your baby is born. Most women find that their heartburn disappears within days, or even hours, after the delivery of their baby.

In the meantime, heartburn can be very distressing. Eating, bending over, even sitting – all can cause pain, whilst at night your sleep may be frequently disturbed. Tell your midwife or doctor how you are feeling, because very occasionally the pain of heartburn may be a sign of more serious illness.

Ideas to try

❏ Avoid eating and drinking at the same time. This may stop your stomach becoming too full.

❏ Try eating six small meals, instead of two or three larger ones. You may find it helps to return to the pattern of eating that helped with pregnancy sickness – little and often. The list of 'Nutritious snacks' on page 75 may give you some ideas.

❏ Avoid fatty foods. These are digested slowly and so keep your stomach full for longer.

❏ Try to avoid spicy foods, coffee and alcohol. These make heartburn worse for many women.

❏ Listen to your body and follow your instincts! Some women find that fizzy drinks make their heartburn worse – others find they help. Similarly, some women find that milk foods make things worse, while others find that milk and plain yoghurts help to ease heartburn.

❏ Try bending your knees and crouching to pick things up, instead of bending over. Keep your back straight and head up. Good practice for picking up small children later on – and much better for your back.

❏ Try to avoid a large meal late at night. You may find it helps to sleep propped up on plenty of firm pillows. Alternatively, try putting a couple of bricks under the feet at the head of your bed to raise it slightly. This may help keep gastric acids in your stomach.

❏ Talk with your midwife or doctor about tablets or medicine to relieve heartburn. The drug they prescribe will probably be an antacid – a special medicine designed to neutralise any gastric acid leaking from your stomach. Antacids will ease the burning sensation in your oesophagus but will not actually stop the escape of acid. This will stop quite naturally and quickly after your baby is born.

❏ There are a number of herbal and homoeopathic remedies for heartburn. Some women have found taking garlic capsules useful, for example. Various shiatsu and osteopathic techniques may also be of help. Like conventional (medical) drugs, complementary medicines and treatments may harm you or your baby if used incorrectly – so do consult a qualified practitioner.

Constipation

'I'd never been constipated in my life before – I didn't know what to do! I thought I already ate a high-fibre diet – but a few dried apricots or figs every day got me back to normal.'

'I've started to drink more water. I'm much less constipated now.'

Constipation means difficulty opening your bowels. When finally passed, the faeces may be unusually small or hard. Being constipated is often associated with haemorrhoids (piles). These are soft, itchy or painful swellings around the anus (back passage). They are made worse by straining to open your bowels, and may sometimes bleed when you have a bowel motion. Constipation during pregnancy is very common; at least one woman in every two will feel constipated at some time.

The pregnancy hormone progesterone is once again partially to blame. Progesterone slows down the natural movement of the bowel. Later on, your growing uterus pushes and squeezes your intestines. Taking less exercise than usual can also slow things down. All of these things mean that waste products take longer than normal to travel through the bowel and so become harder and drier – and more difficult to pass.

Relieving constipation by adding fibre to your diet

❏ Eat a balanced diet with plenty of wholegrain cereals and breads, fruit and vegetables. Dried fruit can help – apricots, prunes and figs eaten raw or stewed, or in crumbles and pies. Or try prune juice or apricot purée with yoghurt or breakfast cereal. Fibrous vegetables, such as carrots and parsnips, may also be useful.

❏ Try rye crispbreads, or a higher-fibre white bread, if you don't like wholemeal bread. Check and compare the nutritional information on the labels.

❏ Eat wholegrain breakfast cereals. It is better to eat these than sprinkle extra bran onto other cereals – doing this can stop your body absorbing valuable nutrients.

❏ Choose brown rice and pasta.

❏ Eat the skin of fruits such as apples and pears.

❏ Lightly scrape, rather than thickly peel, young potatoes and carrots. Try baked potatoes 'in their jackets' (skins). Yam, plantain and cassava are also rich in fibre.

❏ Enjoy tinned baked beans – an excellent and very convenient source of fibre.

❏ Try adding haricot or kidney beans to casseroles to replace some of the meat – cheaper, more fibre and just as nutritious!

Other things to try

❑ Aim to drink 2–3 pints of water, fruit or herbal tea, or other low-sugar drinks – in addition to your usual tea, coffee and milk.

❑ Think about the amount of tea you drink. Some women find that too much strong tea can have a constipating effect.

❑ Give yourself time to go to the toilet. Some women find it difficult in a busy day to visit the toilet when they feel the urge to open their bowels. Delaying going to the toilet can contribute to constipation.

❑ Keep active. Regular exercise that you enjoy – brisk walking, swimming, dancing – can all help relieve constipation.

❑ Talk with your midwife or doctor about any iron tablets or other supplements you are taking. Some iron preparations can make constipation worse. Your midwife or doctor may be able to suggest an alternative tablet or medicine. Or, you may feel you can increase the amount of iron in your diet and reduce the dose of iron tablets. Talk this over with your midwife or doctor.

❑ Talk with your midwife, doctor or pharmacist if you have a problem with piles. They know that it is not unusual for pregnant women to have piles, and will suggest a suitable ointment to relieve the swelling and discomfort.

❑ Some women get relief from constipation through complementary therapies such as reflexology, massage, aromatherapy and shiatsu techniques. Seek advice from a qualified practitioner.

Trying these ideas should relieve your constipation. If they do not, consult your midwife or doctor. She may recommend or prescribe a gentle laxative for you to use for a short time. Some laxatives can be harmful during pregnancy, so always ask for advice from your midwife, doctor or pharmacist before you buy or take one.

It can be difficult

- ❏ Disabled women, or women with a long-term illness, may find pregnancy particularly challenging.
- ❏ Some women find that, whatever they eat, they do not put on much weight. You may worry now that you are pregnant about meeting your baby's nutritional needs. If you can't eat as well as you would like to, it may be a good idea to take a daily multivitamin and mineral supplement. (Check that the vitamin A content is no higher than 600µg.) If your appetite is small or you aren't able to eat much at each sitting, it may help to have three or four small meals with snacks or milky drinks between meals.
- ❏ Other women know that they need to be careful about the energy content of their diet, because they are unable to take much exercise. It is important to eat foods that supply you with all the nutrients needed by you and your baby without too much extra energy. Follow the

basic healthy eating guidelines, taking particular care to choose foods low in fat and sugar.

❑ You may already be able to share a lot of household tasks. If not, now may be the time to organise some help. What support can family and friends give? Are you getting all the benefits and help from social services to which you are entitled? Are there any specialist organisations you can contact now for advice and support?

Many women find some of the side effects of pregnancy hard – but close attention to what you are eating and drinking often help.

Key points

❑ 80% of pregnant women suffer pregnancy sickness in the early months. Take it one day at a time – things generally get better as time goes by. Normal pregnancy sickness will not harm your baby, but see your doctor or midwife if you cannot even drink water.

❑ Relieve pregnancy sickness by eating little and often. Eat whatever your appetite suggests. Pregnancy sickness may be nature's way of telling you to eat more – not less. Rest as much as you can. Do not take any medicines or special foods without asking your midwife or doctor.

❑ Reduce heartburn by eating small, frequent meals. Different things work for different people. Try avoiding coffee, fatty foods and spicy meals. Avoid eating late at night. Your midwife or doctor may prescribe an antacid medicine.

❑ Ease constipation by adding more roughage to your diet. Drink 2–3 pints of water, and try to keep active. Do not take laxative without asking your midwife or doctor. If you are troubled by piles, ask your midwife, doctor or pharmacist to recommend a suitable ointment.

❑ Many women find alternative therapies (such as acupuncture and reflexology) helpful. Seek advice from a qualified practitioner. Don't forget to ask about the cost. Always tell anybody treating or advising you that you are pregnant.

5

Eating for two?

By the time you are three months' pregnant, your baby is basically fully formed – but still only the size of a pear. She can move freely, and can suck and swallow. Blood is flowing around her tiny body, and her kidneys are making urine. She already has little fingernails, and soon her bones will start getting harder.

From now on, your baby will get steadily bigger and stronger. Her internal organs (heart, lungs, kidneys, gut and so on) will continue to develop and prepare for life outside your womb. Her brain will soon begin to grow rapidly, and will continue to grow after she is born and throughout the early years of her life.

Many women find that by the time they are four months' pregnant, they are beginning to feel less sick and tired. You may feel that you can now begin to enjoy being pregnant and can start to plan for the birth of your baby. Around this time, you will probably start to look bigger and, sooner or later, you will feel your baby move inside your womb. You and your midwife will begin to watch the growth of your baby, and you will probably put on more weight as your body prepares an extra store of body fat.

In this chapter we talk about weight changes during pregnancy – why these changes happen, what they mean, and the continuing importance of eating a balanced diet. We also mention the problems that may be caused by starting pregnancy if you are either over- or underweight.

'How much should I be eating?'

'One week she said I'd put on too much weight – then the next she said I wasn't putting on enough. I didn't know what to do!'

It is impossible to say exactly what each and every pregnant woman needs to eat because we all have different nutritional needs. Some women start pregnancy overweight; others are underweight and need to 'catch up'. Some are very active; others find that their instincts are to slow down and rest. Some women will be pregnant with twins (or more), while others will be breastfeeding an older baby. Younger mothers may be still growing, and their energy requirements will be greater. Finally, the nutritional needs of all mothers vary from month to month during their pregnancy; for example, you need more energy in the last few months of pregnancy than at the beginning.

When you are pregnant you do not have to consciously decide how much food to eat. Your appetite is usually the best guide to what you and your growing baby need at each stage of pregnancy.

Some women may find 'eating to appetite' harder than others. Remember that eating very sugary foods may confuse your appetite by causing abrupt swings in the level of sugar in your blood. And eating very fatty foods may mean that you quickly take in large quantities of calories before your appetite has time to catch up.

The key to eating to appetite during pregnancy is the same as at other times: eat plenty of carbohydrates, lots of fruit and vegetables, a moderate amount of protein, and just small quantities of sugar and fat.

It's not just fat . . .

A few women (usually those overweight at the start of pregnancy) may only put on a few kilograms during pregnancy. Their existing stores of body fat are used to meet the needs of pregnancy. On the other hand, some women (usually those underweight at the start of pregnancy) may gain as much as 23kg as their babies grow and their body stores are built up. Both groups of women are likely to give birth to healthy babies of normal weight.

Most pregnant women find that their weight gain during pregnancy lies somewhere between these two groups of women. Average weight gain seems to be between 8kg and 15kg – but there is no 'ideal' weight gain.

Baby

The weight that you will have gained by the end of pregnancy is the sum of several different things. About 7.5kg will be directly related to your baby and her needs:

❏ the weight of her body
❏ her placenta
❏ the fluid in which she floats
❏ extra muscle to strengthen the walls of your uterus
❏ the extra blood your body needs to nourish your baby
❏ new milk-producing cells as your breasts prepare for feeding.

Extra fluid

At least a further 1.5kg of weight will be due to extra body fluid. For many women it will be a lot more than 1.5kg.

This extra fluid is a normal and healthy part of pregnancy. (It seems that women with a moderate amount of fluid retention generally have bigger babies.) Extra fluid in the tissues of your vagina and cervix (neck of the womb) softens these parts ready for giving birth. The joints of your pelvis also become looser, and your nipples get stretchy, ready for breastfeeding. Some of this extra fluid can be seen in swollen feet, ankles, hands, tummy and face. The medical word for this swelling is oedema.

Most women carry about 2 litres of extra fluid by the end of pregnancy. A few may carry as much as 8 litres. This, too, is usually quite normal – but imagine the weight of this amount of bottled water!

There is nothing you can do about the amount of extra fluid in your body. Neither drinking less water nor taking less salt will make a difference. Both actions may, in fact, be harmful.

Sometimes oedema may be a sign of pre-eclampsia, a pregnancy illness that can be very dangerous for you and your baby. The main sign of pre-eclampsia is high blood pressure. All pregnant women should have their blood pressure checked regularly. Other signs of pre-eclampsia include headaches that won't go away, blurred vision, spots in front of your eyes, and pain below your ribs. Pre-eclampsia can develop very quickly. If you are worried, contact your midwife or doctor urgently.

Energy stores

The rest of the weight you may gain is stored as body fat — extra padding on your hips, thighs and tummy. These fat stores are very important. Your baby needs more energy as she grows rapidly during the last three months of pregnancy — but this is just the time when you may find it hard to eat large quantities of food as your growing uterus pushes up against your stomach. This is when your fat stores start to come in useful as your body changes some of the fat into energy to help nourish your baby. You may notice a slight decrease in your weight just before your baby is born. This is normal.

Your body continues to use up your stores of fat after your baby is born. Whether or not you breastfeed her, some of your extra padding will be used to help meet your energy needs during the busy months of caring for a young baby. (We talk more about losing weight in Chapter 8.)

'What is a good weight for me?'

Many things influence how we feel about our bodies. Deciding what is the best weight for each of us can be confusing. This is why it may be helpful to work out your personal Body Mass Index (BMI) – based on your weight before you became pregnant.

Working out your BMI

Your BMI is your weight in kilograms, divided by your height in metres squared (times itself). For example, imagine that you are 1.7m tall and weigh 65kg:

$1.7 \times 1.7 = 2.89$

$65 \div 2.89 = 22.5$

Your BMI is therefore 22.5.

What your BMI means

❑ Less than 20: underweight
❑ 20–25: normal weight
❑ More than 25: overweight

Note: it doesn't matter whether you are 'big boned' or 'petite'. Each of these groups includes a range of BMI figures to allow for different builds.

'I feel I might be overweight'

'After my first was born I'd pick at food, eat the baby's leftovers, and I just didn't lose the weight. Then I fell pregnant again and I had heartburn all the time. Eating helped to keep it at bay, and I gained more than I should have done. I ended up three stone more than I had been.'

If your pre-pregnant Body Mass Index was high (over 25), and you have continued to put on weight during pregnancy, you may be concerned that you are overweight. Talk about this with your doctor or midwife – your weight increase may be due to extra fluid, rather than extra fat.

You may be told that being overweight can cause problems during pregnancy. Although these warnings may sometimes be correct, there is probably not much that you should do about your weight at this time. Scientific research suggests that trying to lose weight during pregnancy does not actually reduce your risk of pregnancy problems. In fact, severely restricting your intake of energy foods ('dieting') may even be harmful to your baby. Dieting during early pregnancy may leave both you and your baby short of vital nutrients – and dieting later on may reduce her birthweight.

This does not mean that your weight is now out of your control. Following the guidelines for a balanced diet and cutting down on sugary and fatty foods can make a big difference. Fill the gaps with fruit and vegetables, and starchy foods like bread, potatoes and pasta. You may find it helpful to read again the sections about fats and sugars in Chapter 1.

Some women find themselves eating an unbalanced diet in response to changes in their lives caused by their pregnancy. You may have stopped work and have time to fill. You may have financial worries or health concerns. You may see pregnancy as a time when you can relax and eat as much as you like, especially if you have spent many years eating carefully and trying to stay slim. Some women find that when they stop smoking (knowing that this is best for themselves and their babies), they start eating an unbalanced diet. In fact, most of us, at some time or another, eat too much of the wrong foods, because we're lonely, bored or anxious. It may help to talk things over with a member of your family, a friend, your family doctor or your midwife. There may be some changes you can make to your life to make it easier to eat a healthy diet.

Weighing scales and pregnancy

Some women find that they are weighed every time they visit their midwife or doctor. Others will be weighed only at their first visit, although women who are overweight or underweight at this visit may be weighed more often. Most experts now feel that it is not necessary to routinely weigh women whose weight was normal at the start of pregnancy. If you are weighed at every visit, you may like to ask your midwife for her reasons.

In any case, weighing during pregnancy is not always very accurate. The scales at the hospital clinic may be different to those at your GP's surgery. You may be wearing different clothes at each visit; a thick pullover and jeans will weigh a lot more than a light summer dress. Finally, remember that every woman's weight – pregnant or not pregnant – varies by at least 1kg from day to day. A lot will depend, for example, on whether you have recently had a large meal or been to the toilet.

'I am worried that my baby isn't growing'

'With both my babies the midwife said I was small at around 34 weeks. I was really worried. In the end, my babies were nearly eight pounds.'

Women themselves are often the best judges of how well their babies are growing – but it is easy to become confused and concerned by things other people say.

If you are weighed regularly during pregnancy and your weight gain seems to slow down or stop, you – or your midwife – may become anxious. The box opposite, 'Weighing scales and pregnancy', explains why weighing is not always accurate. Talk about this with your midwife; together you may be able to get a clearer picture of your weight changes. Remember that many women, especially those with severe pregnancy sickness, may not start to really put on weight until the second half of pregnancy. And women who are overweight at the start of pregnancy may not put on much weight at all.

You and your midwife may decide together that a series of ultrasound scans are needed to measure your baby's growth – although even scans are not always accurate. Scans, however, are generally a more accurate way of assessing your baby's size than palpation (feeling your baby through your tummy) by a midwife or doctor.

If you are still worried, it may be a good idea to think carefully about what you are eating. You may like to keep an 'eating diary' for a few days, writing down everything you eat and drink in a small notebook. Perhaps you could then re-read the first two chapters of this book, and use the guidelines to check how balanced your own diet is. Are you eating five or six servings of starchy foods and at least five servings of fruit and vegetables? Are you listening to your appetite and eating to satisfy your hunger?

Remember that some women find that their appetite is not always a good guide to how much they should be eating. If you have been in the habit of ignoring feelings of hunger and going without food, your appetite may be dulled to the extent that it is no longer a true guide to your needs. Some women are very alarmed by the natural and healthy weight gain of pregnancy, and may restrict what they eat, although they may not realise that this is what they are doing. Could this be you?

Your baby's birthweight

Scientific research has shown that if you enjoy your food, and are eating a full and balanced diet, forcing yourself to eat more will not increase your baby's birthweight. Other things influence your baby's weight: hereditary and racial factors (how much did you weigh as a baby?), the health of your baby's placenta – and smoking. You cannot change the first two things but, you can change smoking habits. We talk more about smoking in Chapter 6.

Specialist help

Certain women may also need extra advice and support:

❑ a very small number of women find that pregnancy sickness continues during pregnancy

❑ young mothers – aged 18 years or less – are still growing themselves and may need special advice

❑ a few women have a medical illness, maybe a thyroid gland problem, which affects their weight

❑ some women have several babies within a few years; their bodies may not have time to recover between pregnancies and their stores of nutrients may be low (most doctors and midwives recommend a minimum of 18 months between giving birth and becoming pregnant again)

Pregnancy and eating disorders

Many women feel they need to control the food they eat so that they do not become overweight. Sometimes this control begins to interfere with a woman's physical and mental health. There are two main types of eating disorder:

❑ anorexia is a total lack of appetite following compulsive restriction of the amount and type of food eaten, sometimes to the point of starvation

❑ bulimia is compulsive 'binge eating' (too much food, all at once) alternating with very restricted eating, sometimes with self-induced vomiting.

The natural increase of appetite during pregnancy, and normal changes in body shape, can be very disturbing to a woman suffering (or recovering from) anorexia or bulimia. Alternatively, pregnancy can sometimes trigger these illnesses in women who were very concerned about their weight before they became pregnant.

Some pregnant women with anorexia or bulimia may struggle against gaining weight during pregnancy, or may begin to lose weight. Other women will find that pregnancy marks the beginning of recovery from their illness.

Women who are severely underweight during pregnancy, and who are not eating enough, are more likely than others to have a baby who is small and weak at birth. This can have long-term effects on your baby's health. If you are worried about putting on weight during pregnancy, talk with your midwife or doctor. A dietitian or specialist counsellor will be able to help.

Going without food during pregnancy

Some pregnant women fast during the daytime throughout Ramadan, for 25 hours during Yom Kippur and Tisha Be'Av, or for other religious, cultural or personal reasons. A healthy baby, inside a healthy and well-nourished mother, will not usually be harmed if her mother has nothing to eat or drink for a day. Drink frequently the day before you start the fast, rest as much as possible during the fast, and break your fast with food full of nutrients and energy such as milk, yoghurt or fruit.

It is not safe to fast for too long, or too often, during pregnancy. This is because sudden and severe changes in your metabolism may affect the health of your developing baby. (Metabolism means the way in which our bodies use food.) If you are unsure what is safe to do, consult your midwife or doctor, and, if appropriate, your religious leader. You may not have to fast if you are not well.

Illness

Some women will be forced to go without food because they fall ill during pregnancy – perhaps through food poisoning or 'flu. If you do not eat for longer than 24 hours, you will probably begin to feel unwell. This is because the way in which your body uses food changes during pregnancy, and a fall in your blood sugar is more likely to cause sickness, giddiness and fainting than at other times. Eventually your body will begin to burn up some of your stores of fat to produce energy. So long as you have good stores of energy and nutrients, your baby will receive nourishment, but you yourself may feel increasingly unwell. If you are still unable to eat solid food, it is important that you try nourishing drinks – milk, juice, soup or sugar water.

Going without water for longer than 12 hours is much more dangerous than going without food. However sick or ill you feel, you must try to take sips of water (ideally water to which a sprinkle of salt and a few spoons of sugar have been added). If you are unable to drink at all, you will become dehydrated (too dry), especially if you have a fever. Eventually this may cause damage to your kidneys or may thicken your blood, increasing your risk of thrombosis (clots in your veins). If you cannot take water, call your family doctor urgently, or ask somebody to take you to the Accident and Emergency Department at your local hospital.

Planning a pregnancy?

Being overweight during pregnancy can cause several problems. (Overweight means a Body Mass Index of more than 25.) You may find that you are more breathless and tired than you would otherwise be. Backache can be particularly troublesome, and you have a greater chance of developing high blood pressure. Having high blood pressure may mean that your baby is born too early.

There is also a link between being overweight and developing 'gestational diabetes', which can cause other problems for you and your baby. (We talk more about this later in this chapter.) Finally, some experts think that women who start pregnancy overweight may find it harder to lose weight after the birth, and may develop a long-term weight problem.

Women who are severely underweight (BMI of 20 or less), or who exercise a lot, may find it hard to conceive. Starting a pregnancy when underweight can also cause problems. If you are only slightly underweight, but you feel that this is normal and know that you enjoy a full and balanced diet – don't worry. On the other hand, if you have been fighting to keep your weight low for some time, and have been restricting what you eat, your body stores of nutrients may be very small. This may increase your risk of anaemia during pregnancy.

Being underweight also increases the chance of your baby being born prematurely (before she is ready), and being weak and small. This can have a long-term effect on her health.

Try to eat a wide range of foods, as described in Chapter 1. If your appetite is small, choose concentrated energy foods, such as dried fruit, nuts, meat, cheese and other dairy products. Talk things over with your GP. A dietitian can give you advice and support to help you get ready for pregnancy.

Gestational (pregnancy) diabetes

During pregnancy your metabolism adapts to make sure that your baby gets all the energy she needs to develop and grow. Although these changes help your baby, extra strain is put on an important part of your digestive system – your pancreas. The pancreas produces a chemical called insulin. Insulin controls the way in which our bodies use glucose (the most basic form of sugar).

People with the condition called 'diabetes' do not produce enough insulin, or insulin might be present but it may not work properly. If they are not treated, the level of glucose in their blood gets higher and higher, leading to a number of serious health problems.

Some people develop diabetes early on. Others become diabetic as they get older, or during a time when their pancreas is under particular strain, such as pregnancy. During pregnancy, your pancreas has to work extra hard to keep up with the needs of your baby. Your pregnancy hormones also add to the strain by reducing the effectiveness of insulin so that your pancreas is required to make even more insulin. For most pregnant women, this causes no problems. A very few (less than one woman in 100) will develop gestational (pregnancy) diabetes.

Most affected pregnant women find that things get back to normal once their babies are born, but a few will continue to need long-term treatment for diabetes. About half of all women who become diabetic during pregnancy and then recover, find that they develop diabetes once again as they get older.

How our bodies use glucose

Let's imagine that we have just eaten a bowl of cereal for breakfast. The bits of cereal are digested (broken down into tiny bits) in the stomach, and travel through the digestive system where glucose and other important nutrients pass into the blood. (The rest of the cereal moves on down into the gut, leaving the fibre to travel down through the large bowel, so keeping everything moving smoothly.) Meanwhile, the pancreas reacts to the presence of glucose and secretes insulin into the blood. The insulin meets up with the glucose and acts as a sort of chemical key, allowing the body to use the glucose, or to change it into fat for storage.

Checking for gestational diabetes

There is a lot of debate among doctors about whether to diagnose and treat gestational diabetes. Some think that if diabetes during pregnancy is not controlled, it can cause problems to both mother and baby. One of the main problems is that the baby may grow particularly big, which can lead to difficulties with her birth. Other doctors believe that so-called gestational diabetes is not necessarily an abnormal condition (although 'true' diabetes should, of course, be diagnosed and treated).

In some areas, all mothers are tested for gestational diabetes; in other places you will only be tested if you are felt to be at increased risk of developing gestational diabetes. Your risk may be greater if:

❑ you are overweight
❑ you have had a large baby already
❑ you have family members with diabetes
❑ you have high blood pressure
❑ you are aged over 35 years.

A diagnosis of diabetes is usually made following a series of blood glucose tests. If your doctor thinks that you have diabetes, you will be told how the condition can be controlled. (There is no 'cure' for diabetes − no way of making it 'go away'; the aim of treatment is to stop your blood glucose levels from going too high and causing further health problems.)

Treatment

All women with gestational diabetes will be told about changes that they can make to their diet to help control their blood glucose levels. A dietitian, or specialist diabetes nurse, should be available to give detailed advice. Ask as many questions as you wish, and make sure you have information in writing to share with your partner or family. As well as making changes to their diet, some women will be advised to have regular injections of insulin.

If you have gestational diabetes, you will be asked to return to the hospital at frequent intervals, so that your blood glucose levels can be checked. Some women find that making so many visits causes financial problems and other difficulties. Talk the situation over with your midwife; there may be some kind of help available.

Glucose in your urine

You may be told during pregnancy that you have glucose in your urine. This does not mean that you have diabetes. Your kidneys work much harder during pregnancy, and this may cause some 'leaking' of glucose into your urine. This happens for many pregnant women (and is one reason that you are more likely to develop yeast infections such as thrush during pregnancy). Diabetes can only be properly diagnosed following a number of blood tests.

Diabetes and your diet

Please note! These are simple guidelines only. An expert should give you detailed and individual advice. The three basic principles of a diabetic diet are:

- ❏ Follow the guidelines for a balanced diet (as described in Chapter 1).
- ❏ Eat and drink regularly during the day, so that your blood glucose levels stay relatively stable – neither too low, nor too high. This may mean smaller main meals and one or two extra snacks. Foods containing soluble fibre (such as oats, beans, peas, lentils and some fruits) are more slowly absorbed than others and so help to avoid sudden rises in blood glucose. For this reason, many diabetic women find that low-sugar muesli and porridge make good breakfast foods.
- ❏ Avoid large intakes of sugar, either in food or drink, since your pancreas may not be able to produce enough insulin to deal with it. Remember that the higher that the word 'sugar' appears on a list of ingredients, the greater the sugar content of that food. Particularly to be avoided are the rapidly absorbed sugars 'dextrose', 'glucose', 'sucrose' and 'maltose'. The natural sugars in milk ('lactose') and fruit ('fructose') are absorbed more slowly. Replace sugary foods with starchy foods, as described in Chapter 1.

Everybody's metabolism is different. Many women can control their gestational diabetes by paying careful attention to their diet; others will need extra help from regular insulin injections. Talk with your doctor, midwife or consultant about how to manage your diet in pregnancy.

Key points

❏ It is impossible to say how much each pregnant woman should eat. Every woman is different, with unique needs. The key is to eat to appetite, following the basic plan for healthy eating.

❏ There is no 'ideal' weight gain during pregnancy. The weight of your baby is only a part of your total weight gain. Weighing during pregnancy does not accurately reflect the growth of your baby. If you are eating a full and balanced diet, simply eating more food will not increase your baby's weight.

❏ Do not try to lose weight during pregnancy. Eat a balanced diet, filling gaps with fruit, vegetables and starchy carbohydrates, rather than sugary or fatty foods.

❏ If your appetite is small, choose concentrated energy foods, such as meat, dried fruit, nuts, cheese and other dairy produce.

❏ Women with untreated eating disorders (anorexia or bulimia) may have small, weak babies. If you are very worried about putting on weight during pregnancy, talk with your midwife or doctor. A dietitian or specialist counsellor will be able to help.

6

Healthy eating and lifestyle

A balanced diet is central to our physical and mental well-being. This is particularly true during pregnancy when your body is sheltering and nurturing your baby. But some things in our lives can interfere with a balanced eating pattern.

Smoking and alcohol and drug abuse all have a direct effect on your baby and on levels of vital nutrients. They may also have an indirect effect by diverting money – and time – away from caring for ourselves.

In this chapter we outline the dangers to you and your baby, and suggest the steps that we can all take to protect the health of mothers and babies.

Alcohol and pregnancy

'I'd rather someone told me to stop drinking completely. I find it really confusing to be told I can have "a little". What's "a little"?'

Many women in Western society drink alcohol, and most do so sensibly. Alcohol drunk in moderation, with consideration for others and respect for ourselves, can add to life's pleasures.

Alcohol and your baby

Pregnancy is a time to be particularly careful. Heavy drinking during pregnancy can damage your baby, as well as yourself. Alcohol crosses the placenta to your baby very easily and quickly. Too much alcohol on a regular basis during pregnancy may cause a condition called 'fetal alcohol syndrome'. ('Fetal' refers to the baby, and 'syndrome' means a collection of problems.)

Babies with fetal alcohol syndrome tend to grow slowly, before and after they are born. They may have problems with their sight or hearing, and later learning difficulties. Some are born with cleft palates, a condition in which a baby's mouth is not properly developed.

Pregnant women who drink more than 6 units of alcohol each day during pregnancy have a high chance of having a baby with fetal alcohol syndrome. Out of every 50 women who drink this heavily during pregnancy, between one and 12 of their babies will have fetal alcohol syndrome. Women who drink between 2 and 6 units of alcohol each day may give birth to babies with a milder form of fetal alcohol syndrome. It is not yet clear from research exactly how much alcohol you can drink before your baby is harmed. Smoking, a poor diet and the use of illegal drugs all increase the chance of a baby being affected by fetal alcohol syndrome.

How much is too much?

While you are pregnant (or planning to get pregnant) you should certainly not drink more than 1 or 2 units of alcohol once or twice a week. Try not to have more than 2 units of alcohol in a single day. The type of drink makes no difference – it is the total amount of alcohol (measured in units) that matters. (Check the chart over the page.)

Many women decide to give up alcohol altogether – either because they suddenly dislike the taste, or they feel that no alcohol at all is the only absolutely safe thing to do during pregnancy.

Units of alcohol

1 unit of alcohol =
1 pub measure ('single' or 25ml) of spirits
1 pub glass of wine (100ml)
Half a pint of ordinary strength beer or lager
Quarter of a pint of strong beer or cider
1 sherry glass of sherry, port, vermouth (55ml)
(1 unit of alcohol = 10g of alcohol)

Remember that home measures of wine or spirits tend to be a lot more generous than pub measures. Measure out a unit of alcohol in millilitres into a glass at home and use that as your guide. Brands of wines, beer and lager vary a lot in the amount of alcohol they contain. Check the 'alcohol % vol.' label on bottles and cans and choose the lowest. Try alcohol-free and low-alcohol wines and beers.

'I didn't know I was pregnant'

Many women worry that episodes of heavy drinking or drunkenness early in pregnancy may have caused harm. If you are generally healthy and well nourished, there is very little chance that your baby will have been harmed by heavy drinking on one or two occasions.

Drinking less alcohol

'I feel so left out not being able to drink. It's made me realise how much I depended on alcohol to enjoy things.'

It may not always be easy to reduce the amount of alcohol you drink – but the dangers of not doing so are very real. Both your health and your baby's health are at risk. Reducing your intake of alcohol to a safe level would be an enormous positive contribution towards your baby's future wellbeing. It is a contribution that you alone can make.

You may find some of these ideas helpful:

❏ quench your thirst with non-alcoholic drinks
❏ sip your drink, and put your glass down between sips
❏ try alcohol-free or low-alcohol drinks
❏ ask family and friends to support you by not offering to pour or prepare drinks
❏ find other ways to help you relax – a warm bath, lovemaking, music, watching television
❏ keep some days of the week alcohol-free.

If you have been used to drinking a lot, and find it hard to reduce the amount you drink during pregnancy, you probably need extra help. Women can get addicted to alcohol, as they can to smoking or certain drugs. You can overcome this addiction – but most people need specialist support to do so. Talk with your midwife or doctor – or one of the national telephone helplines. Contact details for organisations that help with alcohol problems are listed at the end of this book.

Alcohol and you

Pregnant or not, drinking too much alcohol can damage almost every part of the body including digestive system, heart and circulation, and brain and nervous system. Women who use alcohol increase their risk of breast cancer and liver disease. Both can kill. Too much alcohol alters the metabolism, interferes with the storage of nutrients and dulls the appetite. Women who drink heavily are often very short of vital nutrients such as folic acid, B group vitamins, vitamin A, zinc, magnesium and iron. Alcohol is full of 'empty calories'; it has no nutritional value, and can contribute to an unhealthy weight gain.

Women who drink too much alcohol come from all sections of society. At-risk groups include:

❏ adolescent women
❏ career-oriented single women under the age of 25
❏ divorced and separated women.

Many women who abuse alcohol try to convince themselves that they do not have a problem. Others may hide their problem from other people. Many women find it hard to ask for help and support to stop drinking alcohol.

Women cannot tolerate alcohol as well as some men, because of differences in body size and metabolism. Women who are not pregnant (or planning to become pregnant) should drink no more than 14–21 units of alcohol a week, and should aim to keep one or two days alcohol-free.

Smoking – you know the risks!

'I gave up smoking completely. It was the natural thing to do. I just didn't want it.'

'I just couldn't give up, but I cut it down to just one a day.'

Although smoking is enjoyed by many people, it is a cruel and dangerous addiction. Most women nowadays are aware of the harm that smoking can do to themselves and to their babies – but knowing the risks may not make giving up smoking any easier.

Apart from increasing her risk of lung cancer and heart attacks, a woman who smokes is more likely to develop cancer of the cervix. Overall, smoking accounts for a third of all deaths of middle-aged people.

A pregnant woman who smokes is not only harming herself. She is also damaging her baby. A baby born to a smoker is:

❑   more likely than other babies to be abnormal in some way
❑   twice as likely to be born prematurely
❑   more likely to suffer from placenta problems around the time of birth
❑   three times more likely to be underweight at birth (even if she is born on time)
❑   more likely to be a victim of 'cot death'.

Smoking – how it harms your baby

Your baby needs oxygen to live and grow. Oxygen passes from your lungs into your blood, where it combines with haemoglobin. Haemoglobin carries oxygen to your placenta, where it passes through into your baby's circulation. Each time you smoke a cigarette, you breathe in a gas called carbon monoxide. This gas interferes with the transport of oxygen by your haemoglobin, and your baby's supply of oxygen is reduced. Without a good supply of oxygen, your baby's growth may be stunted.

Other chemicals in cigarettes cause further harm. Nicotine narrows the blood vessels in your placenta, and this reduces the amount of oxygen and nutrients flowing to your baby. Nicotine also makes your baby's heart beat faster. Smokers have lower nutrient intakes than non-smokers, and may be deficient in folic acid, zinc and vitamin C.

Most of these effects are 'dose-related' – the more you smoke, the greater the damage. The damage caused by smoking is quickly reversed when you stop smoking. There is some evidence that smoking cigarettes low in carbon monoxide, nicotine and tar may reduce the effect of smoking on your baby's birthweight.

Smoking and antioxidants

In Chapter 2 we explained the action of antioxidants – special nutrients that help fight the effects of pollutants and other toxic substances. The main antioxidants are vitamins C and E, selenium, zinc and beta carotene.

Antioxidants are especially important for women who smoke – or who cannot avoid smoke from other people's cigarettes. You may like to increase your intake of vitamin C and zinc, in particular. However, although antioxidants may benefit smokers, there is little proof that they reduce the harm caused to babies by cigarette smoke.

Planning a pregnancy?

Both women and men who smoke tend to be less fertile. Heavy smoking also increases your chance of a miscarriage.

Giving up smoking before you become pregnant will give your body time to adjust. Your nutrient levels will recover, and levels of toxic chemicals will fall. You are less likely to put on extra weight if you give up smoking before becoming pregnant.

The best for your baby

Giving up smoking is not easy. For many women, smoking represents a short and temporary escape from the pressures of everyday life. For others, smoking is an important part of their relationship with work colleagues, friends or family. But stopping smoking – or, at least, reducing the number and strength of cigarettes – is a strong and special thing that you can do for your baby. Many things in life are out of our control – but the hand that holds the cigarette you smoke is yours to control.

The sooner you give up smoking, the better it will be for your baby. It is never too late to give up (or cut down). Whatever your stage of pregnancy, the benefits of stopping smoking will be felt immediately by both you and your baby.

Nicotine chewing gum and skin patches

These things help lots of people to give up smoking – but it is not clear if they are safer than smoking in pregnancy. There are many excellent leaflets and other sources of advice and help for women wanting to stop smoking. Ask your midwife about local support groups, or contact one of the national telephone helplines. We give contact details at the end of this book.

'My friend smoked 30 cigarettes a day and gave birth to an 8lb baby'

Your friend was lucky! Researchers have been studying the effects of smoking for many years. Statistics regarding the health of tens of thousands of mothers and babies have been examined. The relationship between maternal smoking and the poor health of babies has been proven many times over. There will always be lucky ones – but not many.

'I think having a small baby would make labour easier'

No – that is not true! Labour with a small baby is not usually any easier for the mother – and it can be a lot harder for the baby. A small baby has less strength to cope with labour. She has a greater risk of dying during labour than other babies. Furthermore, slow growth during pregnancy and being underweight at birth can affect your baby's health well into adulthood.

Drugs and pregnancy

'I know I have to be careful with drugs, but I got quite a shock when my midwife told me that some aromatherapy oils may be harmful too.'

'Drugs' means any kind of tablet, medicine, suppository, inhalant, ointment or oil – whether it is prescribed by a doctor or other practitioner, chosen by you from a pharmacy, or bought illegally ('street' or 'recreational' drugs). We use the term 'drugs' to include all nutritional supplements, herbal preparations, massage and aromatherapy oils, homoeopathic remedies, anything you would take for a headache or for constipation, cough and cold treatments, and caffeine.

Most drugs pass through the placenta and into your baby's blood. Others may change the way your body works in some way – and so have an indirect effect on your baby.

During pregnancy your baby is particularly vulnerable to the effects of drugs taken by you. There are two main reasons for this vulnerability:

❏ your baby's rapidly developing body is very sensitive to poisons in her environment
❏ her liver is not ready to deal with harmful substances entering her body.

Some drugs taken during pregnancy can be beneficial – for example, antibiotics taken by the mother will also help fight infection in her baby. Other drugs will seem to have no effect on the baby (although the results of research, in some cases, may be unclear). A few drugs will cause permanent harm. The 1960s thalidomide tragedy is probably the example that many people remember. A drug taken at this time by mothers to relieve pregnancy sickness caused short or missing arms and legs in their children.

Planning a pregnancy?

> 'I've been on antidepressants for ages. I checked with my doctor – just casually – she said the low dose I was taking was OK if I got pregnant. I'm glad I asked, because I fell pregnant the next month, but I would have been really worried.'

Some women need to continue to take their regular drugs throughout pregnancy to keep themselves physically or mentally healthy – drugs to control epilepsy, diabetes or thyroid problems, blood pressure medication, antidepressants, painkillers, drugs to treat addictions, and so on.

If you take regular drugs such as these, do consult your doctor before you become pregnant so that your drug routine can be looked at carefully, and a balance found between your health and the health of your planned baby. Many drugs may do their greatest harm in the first three months of pregnancy and drug routines can be adapted to take this into account. Some long-term conditions – such as diabetes – need to be carefully controlled during the early weeks of pregnancy.

If this kind of advance planning has not been possible, you must contact your doctor – urgently – as soon as you think you may be pregnant. Do not stop taking your regular drugs until you have spoken with your doctor.

Taking care during pregnancy

❏ Never buy 'over-the-counter' (non-prescription) medicines for yourself without first checking with your pharmacist or doctor. They will be able to recommend alternative drugs or other safe treatments.

❏ Always tell your doctor, pharmacist and any-body else advising you on your health – includ-ing your dentist – that you are pregnant, or planning to become pregnant. They will help you make decisions by balancing your own health needs against the risks of certain drugs to your baby.

❏ Always check with your pharmacist, doctor or a qualified herbalist before taking any herbal medicines or tablets. Fruit and herbal teas sold in supermarkets are generally safe – but be care-ful with preparations brewed by family or friends, or sold in health-food shops.

❏ Always check with your pharmacist, doctor or a qualified practitioner before using any homoeo-pathic remedies, aromatherapy preparations or massage oils.

Drugs of addiction – 'street drugs'

There has not been much research into the effects of street drugs on babies. Many women who use these drugs also smoke, drink alcohol, eat an unbalanced diet and have poor living conditions – so the actual causes of some problems can be unclear. Some drugs may be contaminated with other substances, and these can add to the dangers.

Most drugs increase the risk of your baby being born too early, and being jumpy and difficult to settle during the early weeks. Amphetamines, Ecstasy and cocaine may also cause heart problems in babies. Glue sniffing, amphetamines, Ecstasy and heroin increase your baby's risk of being very small at birth. Cocaine and solvent use can lead to problems with your baby's bladder and kidneys. Cocaine can cause serious blood pressure problems in mothers, and gangrenous toes and fingers in babies. Research is not clear about the effects of LSD on babies born to women who use this drug.

The problems associated with regular cannabis use include:

❏ premature birth
❏ your baby being jumpy and irritable during the first weeks of her life
❏ your baby developing slowly in her early years.

There is no research linking cannabis use by mothers with disability in their babies.

So far, little is known about the effects of drug use on long-term mental development of babies and children.

Some research suggests that damage is not permanent, and children born to women who used street drugs during pregnancy eventually catch up with other children.

Some women are addicted to medical drugs such as tranquillisers and sedatives. The effects of use of these drugs during pregnancy are not yet clear. If you feel that you depend – physically or emotionally – on one of these drugs, you too need sound advice and skilled support to ensure the best for yourself and your baby.

Pregnancy and drugs of addiction

Drug addiction during pregnancy is not uncommon. Across the country, there are a number of specialist maternity departments caring for women who abuse drugs. Many other hospitals have staff specially trained to understand and help meet your needs. Midwives and doctors know that women who abuse drugs during pregnancy need sympathetic support rather than criticism.

Many drug-using women are keen to give up their habit. Experts feel that this is safe and possible during pregnancy, although it is best to have skilled support. Although detoxification is possible at any time during pregnancy, the sooner you do so, the better for your baby. Make contact with a midwife early in your pregnancy by phoning or visiting your nearest maternity unit.

The babies of drug-using mothers do not always have to be cared for in special nurseries. You and your baby need not be separated. Breastfeeding is possible – and best for both you and your baby.

Caffeine

'I love my cups of tea – so I was quite upset when I suddenly went off tea early in pregnancy. But maybe my body was trying to tell me something.'

You need to limit the amount of caffeine you have each day, but you don't have to cut it out completely. Caffeine occurs naturally in a range of foods, such as coffee, tea and chocolate, and it's also added to some soft drinks and 'energy' drinks.

It's important not to have more than 300mg of caffeine a day. This is because high levels of caffeine can result in babies with low birth weight, miscarriage or even stillbirth.

Caffeine may contribute to two other problems:

❑ Caffeine taken with a meal may reduce the amount of iron that your body can absorb from food. Drink your tea or coffee an hour before your meal – or wait two hours afterwards.

❑ Caffeine may cause 'restless leg syndrome', an odd feeling of being unable to keep your legs still. The syndrome tends to worsen during pregnancy. Cutting down on caffeine may relieve the symptoms.

How much caffeine is too much?

Experts suggest a maximum of 300mg caffeine each day. Roughly, 300mg means any of these:

- ❏ 3 mugs of instant coffee (100mg each)
- ❏ 4 cups of instant coffee (75mg each)
- ❏ 3 cups of brewed coffee (100mg each)
- ❏ 6 cups of tea (50mg each)
- ❏ 8 cans of cola (up to 40mg each)
- ❏ 4 cans of 'energy' drink (up to 80mg each)
- ❏ 8 (50g) bars of chocolate (up to 50mg each)

So, if you eat a bar of chocolate and drink three cups of tea, a can of cola and a cup of instant coffee in a day, you'll have reached your 300mg limit.

Remember that caffeine is also found in certain cold and 'flu remedies, so always check with your GP or a health professional before taking any of these.

Decaffeinated coffee has had most of the caffeine removed, although some similar substances may remain.

Cravings and aversions

'I'm a bit worried. I've gone off oranges, lettuce, olives, fish – all the healthy things!'

'I went off garlic with one baby, went off tea and coffee with all of them, but of course I've never stopped liking chocolate!'

Early in pregnancy, many women find that they suddenly dislike the taste and smell of things like alcohol, cigarette smoke and caffeine. Other women detest certain perfumes, petrol fumes, the smell of cooking, fats, red meat – even oranges. At the same time, or maybe a little later in pregnancy, some women develop strong cravings for certain foods like pickled cabbage, anchovies, peppermints.

We do not know for sure why pregnant women develop these cravings and aversions. The hormones of pregnancy may change how things taste and smell. Pregnancy sickness probably plays a part, too. Sometimes women crave certain foods containing nutrients in which they are deficient. Your cultural background may also influence your choices; without deliberately deciding to do so, you may find yourself following a tradition of avoiding or eating certain special foods during pregnancy.

For women across the world, pregnancy is a special time when – maybe for the first time in their lives – they are special to themselves and to others. Asking for certain foods – and refusing others – may be one way of making the most of this special feeling.

Ask yourself if your food likes and dislikes are stopping you eating a balanced diet. If they don't, then you probably need not worry. If you have any doubts, speak with your midwife or doctor.

What is pica?

Pica is a rare condition in which pregnant women want to eat non-food items such as clay, toothpaste, coal, soil and chalk. Pica can be dangerous. Some of the substances eaten may interfere with the body's absorption of minerals, and so lead to malnutrition. Many substances are poisonous. Occasionally, pica can be a sign of a nutritional deficiency or another illness needing medical attention. Consult your midwife or doctor if you crave non-food substances.

For many women, pregnancy can be a time of positive changes. Now may be the time to change to a more balanced (and, ultimately, more satisfying) diet. It may also be the time to make those lifestyle changes that lie within your control. Women want to do the best for their babies. Do the best for yourself as well.

Key points

❏ Heavy drinking can harm you and your baby. Do not drink more than 4 units of alcohol in a week (no more than 2 units in a single day).

❏ Smoking can also harm you and your baby in many ways. It's never too late to stop smoking, or cut down. Both you and your baby will immediately feel the benefits.

❏ Always tell your doctor, pharmacist, dentist (and anybody else advising or treating you) that you are pregnant. Always check with a pharmacist before buying 'over-the-counter' (non-prescription) drugs or alternative remedies (such as herbs and massage oils).

❏ Street drugs, and other drugs of addiction such as tranquillisers and sedatives, can harm you and your baby. Detoxification is possible during pregnancy, and breastfeeding is recommended. Make contact early in pregnancy with a midwife or doctor to get skilled and sympathetic help.

❏ Try not to drink more than 3 mugs of instant coffee or strong tea each day.

7

Questions and (some) answers

'Will my baby be all right?'

'I've read all this about healthy eating – and now I'm really worried! I felt awful for the first three months of my pregnancy so I hardly ate anything. Since then, I've just eaten junk food. Will my baby be all right?'

Until she is born, nobody can say for certain that your baby – or anybody else's baby – will be all right. All we can say is that the vast majority of babies are healthy, even if their mothers have been vomiting a lot during pregnancy and have been unable to eat at all well.

Remember that your body is designed to nurture your baby, both before and after her birth. Your pregnant body is not some delicate piece of machinery, liable to break down and stop as soon as anything goes slightly wrong. Your body is strong and resourceful, and your baby – even when tiny – is a tough little being, determined to live and grow.

Sometimes this determination can be hard for mothers. If, for some reason, you cannot eat a balanced diet, your baby will draw on your body's stores of nutrients to provide for her needs. When these are all finished your fat and muscle will be broken down to release more nutrients. Minerals will be drawn from your bones to help build up your baby's bones. Your baby will grow – but your own resistance to infection will fall, your bones will eventually become weaker, and your body's healing ability will diminish.

If you have had a poor diet for some time, you may now be in urgent need of some nutrients. It may be a good idea to take a multivitamin and mineral supplement for a few weeks. Remember to choose one without vitamin A. Talk with your midwife or doctor.

'Junk' food

As for the junk food – even this contains vital nutrients for you and your baby! The main problem with meals based on so-called junk food is that they are often unbalanced – too much fat and sugar, and not enough of some vitamins and minerals.

Think about what you enjoy eating and how it can fit into a healthy eating plan. Take a pizza, for example: bread dough base, dairy products (cheese topping), protein (cheese and any added meat), vegetables (onions, tomato paste, olives). To make a balanced meal, don't add chips – choose instead a large helping of vegetables – peas, broccoli, sweetcorn – or salad, and a piece of fruit to follow.

In conclusion, remember that other things, beside what you eat, will affect your baby's development and health. Some of these things are outside your control – for example, her genetic background and environmental pollution. Others you can take responsibility for – making sure your blood pressure is regularly checked, cutting down or giving up smoking and alcohol, and preparing yourself for her birth.

'Does fruit have to be fresh?'

'I can't get to the shops every day to buy fresh fruit and vegetables. What should I do?'

Vegetables, in particular, do not have to be fresh to be good. Frozen vegetables, such as peas, beans and sweet-corn, are just as nutritious and are available throughout the year. Tinned vegetables such as tomatoes, baked beans and garden or processed peas are reasonably priced and nutritious. Canned pulses like kidney beans or chick-peas can be eaten cold with salad items, or added to meat casseroles.

Fresh carrots, onions, cabbage, potatoes (and other root vegetables such as sweet potatoes, parsnips and turnips) all keep well if kept covered in a cool place.

Tinned fruit is almost as nutritious as fresh fruit. Choose fruit canned in juice rather than syrup for more flavour and less sugar. And don't forget dried fruit – apricots, dates, raisins and sultanas. Although some nutritional value is lost in the drying process, fruit in this form is still excellent. If you like sweet things, you may find a dried apricot or date a healthy substitute for a piece of chocolate or other sugary treat.

Chapter 1 explains the nutritional importance of vegetables and fruit – and Chapter 2 suggests ways to preserve the vitamins in these foods.

How to grow fresh vegetables – without a garden!

Sprouted seeds contain useful vitamins. All you need is:

❑ mustard and cress seeds, mung beans, aduki beans or alfalfa seeds
❑ a wide-necked jam jar
❑ a small square of muslin (or old tights)
❑ an elastic band.

This is what you do:

1. Overnight, soak a small quantity of the beans or seeds in the jam jar.
2. The next morning, use the elastic band to fix the muslin tightly over the neck of the jar.

3. Fill the jar with water, and then drain all the water out by leaving the jar tilted steeply on its side. The seeds will start to sprout in this position.
4. Leaving the muslin in place, repeat this twice a day. Don't let the plants dry out – or get waterlogged.
5. Eat the sprouts (seeds, beans and all) as soon as they look long enough – don't wait too long!

Cress and alfalfa sprouts are best raw, in salads or sandwiches. Mung and aduki bean sprouts can be eaten raw or cooked. To get rid of the skins of the mung beans, place the sprouts in a bowl of cold water and stir, so that the skins float to the top.

Going to the dentist

'My midwife has told me to make a dentist's appointment. Why?'

Progesterone (one of the pregnancy hormones) helps prepare your body for giving birth. One way in which it does this is to make the connective tissue of your body softer and moister. (Connective tissue is the 'packing' that supports and holds our body parts.) You may notice one side effect of this in your mouth as your gums become softer and slightly swollen.

Because of these changes, your gums are more likely during pregnancy to bleed, become inflamed (sore and red) and get infected. Infected gums can lead, in turn, to tooth decay. Severe infection in one part of the body may affect other parts, and it is possible that some premature births are caused by infection. Regular and thorough teeth cleaning are particularly important during pregnancy.

It is also worth knowing that basic sugars – those found naturally in starchy foods and fruit – are less likely to harm your teeth (and contribute to tooth decay) than sugars added artificially to food and drinks. Remember, too, that the longer any kind of sugar is in contact with your teeth, the greater the risk of damage to your teeth. This is why eating a banana or biscuit followed by a drink of water is better than sucking a sweet or candy bar for 5 or 10 minutes. We talk more about avoiding sugary foods in Chapter 8.

Dental care during pregnancy

Dental care is free during pregnancy, and for the first year after your baby is born, from NHS dentists. Talk with a dentist, or dental hygienist, about the best way to clean your teeth. Your dentist can also check to see if you have any small spots of tooth decay which may need treating. Make sure that your dentist knows you are pregnant so that she or he can decide on the safest method of treatment. Mercury fillings are not recommended during pregnancy.

'Do I need iron tablets?'

'According to my antenatal card, the level of iron in my blood has fallen from 12.5g/dl to 10.5g/dl – but my midwife says I don't need iron tablets. Why not?'

Two or three times during your pregnancy you will be offered a blood test to measure your haemoglobin – the level of iron in your blood. (Haemoglobin is often abbreviated to 'Hb', and is measured in grams per decilitre, written as 'g/dl'.) A healthy non-pregnant woman will have a haemoglobin level between 11.5g/dl and 16.5g/dl.

During pregnancy the amount of plasma (the watery part of the blood) in your body increases to meet the needs of you and your growing baby. This increase means that your blood becomes more dilute, and haemoglobin levels appear to fall. A haemoglobin level as low as 9.0g/dl is quite normal in pregnancy.

This increase in plasma volume and relative drop in haemoglobin are both normal and healthy. Research shows that women whose haemoglobin levels do not adapt in this way are more likely to develop pre-eclampsia and give birth to underweight babies.

Side effects

During pregnancy your body absorbs iron much better than at other times – and the more iron you need, the better your body absorbs it from food. This means that you are unlikely to need iron supplements if you are eating a varied balanced diet including foods rich in iron. Have another look at the list of iron-rich foods (and ways of improving the absorption of iron) in Chapter 2.

Remember that iron tablets can have unpleasant side effects, including sickness and constipation. Iron supplements may also interfere with the absorption of other important nutrients such as zinc.

A few women in the UK do become genuinely anaemic during pregnancy, and this can cause serious problems for both mother and baby. Some women – especially very young women – start pregnancy with low levels of iron. Other women may have low stores following very heavy periods or an unbalanced diet. Anaemia may also be caused by a shortage of other nutrients, such as folic acid. Occasionally anaemia is a sign of a serious blood disorder or other illness.

Checking for anaemia

If anaemia is suspected, your midwife or doctor will advise you to have further blood tests, including assessment of your mean corpuscular volume (MCV). The MCV is a more accurate measure of the amount of iron in your blood than a simple haemoglobin test because it examines the health of individual red blood cells. MCV level during pregnancy is normally 84–99fl. A level less than 84fl may indicate that you are short of iron.

Overseas holiday

'My boyfriend and I are going to Spain for a week when I am six months' pregnant. I'm really worried about things like listeria. What should I do?'

Remember that the majority of food manufacturers, shops, cafes and restaurants, both at home and abroad, are as concerned about food safety as you are – after all, their livelihood depends on staying in business!

Buying food

- ❏ Choose popular eating places with a good turnover of customers – and therefore food.
- ❏ Avoid roadside stalls or kiosks, which may not have adequate cold storage or cooking facilities.
- ❏ Avoid sandwich fillings and other foods that have been prepared and left standing for several hours – things like chicken or tuna in mayonnaise or dressed salads.
- ❏ Say 'no' to all salad ingredients if you have any concerns about the water supply used to wash the ingredients.
- ❏ Wipe or wash fresh fruit before eating, even if it looks clean. If this is not possible, peel fruit.
- ❏ Use a coolbox chilled with an icepack to store food bought in advance for a picnic.
- ❏ In some countries unpasteurised milk is sold. If pasteurised milk is not available or you are otherwise

unsure what you are being offered, it may be better to choose tinned, sterilised, UHT or dried milk.

Choosing a meal

❑ Choose meals that need to be freshly cooked – rather than things like pies or pasties that just need to be reheated, or smoked or cured foods such as Parma ham and pastrami.

❑ Choose simple dishes over fancy foods – especially if you and the waiters share a language problem. A well-cooked beefsteak or piece of fish with plenty of fresh vegetables may be preferable to a complicated seafood dish with unknown ingredients, for example.

❑ Avoid shellfish, since this is a frequent cause of food poisoning.

❑ Avoid dishes made using raw or lightly cooked eggs. Many catering businesses do use pasteurised eggs, but it is hard to be sure.

❑ Take care with grilled or barbecued foods. When the food is on your plate, check that it is cooked through and piping hot before you tuck in.

Please see Chapter 3 for further information about food safety during pregnancy.

Organic food

'Should I be eating organic food now that I'm pregnant?'

Most food in the world is grown with the help of pesticides and herbicides (pest and weed killers), artificial fertilisers and other chemicals and drugs. Experts argue that these chemicals are needed in order to produce enough cheap food to satisfy growing populations. However, many people are now becoming more and more worried about the levels of these potentially toxic chemicals in our environment.

The UK government and food producers are taking action. Some toxic substances have been banned, including DDT (a pesticide) and PCBs (materials widely used in electrical equipment). Levels of both of these in food products are now falling. Restrictions are in place on the amount of dangerous chemicals allowed in our food, but because new chemicals are continually being introduced, regulations cannot always keep up.

A small proportion of our foods still contains potentially dangerous levels of chemicals. We do not know the long-term effects of even low levels of toxic substances in our food and water.

Babies

Babies are particularly vulnerable, both during pregnancy and their first year. This is because they are growing very rapidly and so take in a large amount of food in relation to the small size of their bodies. In addition, their livers are not yet ready to deal with any toxic substances with which they may come into contact. While inside you, your baby is partially protected, but once born she will be exposed to chemicals in milk and other foods.

Breastmilk

Although – like artificial baby milk – your breast-milk will contain traces of some chemicals, the presence of these is far outweighed by the amazing ability of human milk to protect your baby against infections and other illnesses, both immediately and later in her life. Breastfeeding is, without any doubt, the best and most natural way to feed your baby.

Some women feel that it is safer to try to avoid what chemicals they can by using organic foods. Organic food is food produced without the use of artificial chemicals. For example, organic fruit and vegetables are grown in orchards and fields that have not been sprayed or fertilised with artificial chemicals, and organic bread is made from wheat grown in similar conditions. Organic meat and dairy produce are from animals that have grazed on grass grown with natural fertilisers, and have eaten only fodder free from drugs and other chemicals.

The main problem with buying organic food is the

increased cost compared to non-organic items. Prices are gradually falling, but even so, some vegetables and fruit may be twice the cost of normal produce. Organic bread and dairy produce in larger supermarkets tend to be cheaper – but are still more expensive than the cheapest brands available.

Organic food – meeting the cost

You could:

❏ consider the regular use of just one or two organic foods – maybe basic items such as milk or bread

❏ find out about local organic vegetable box schemes – a guaranteed supply at guaranteed prices

❏ look out for market stalls or farm shops specialising in organic produce

❏ grow some vegetables of your own (see our section about sprouting seeds earlier in this chapter)

❏ tell your local greengrocer or supermarket manager that you want to buy their organic food – but it is too expensive (we hope that public opinion will eventually help increase supplies and reduce costs)

The problem with peanuts

'I've heard that pregnant and breastfeeding women shouldn't eat peanuts. Is this true?'

Peanut allergy is a real and increasing problem. One in every 200 four-year-old children is now allergic to peanuts. Most of those suffering from peanut allergy develop the problem before their third birthday. Although some children seem to eventually grow out of peanut allergy, for others the problem will remain for life.

An allergy is an over-sensitive response to a specific substance, causing skin problems, wheezing, tightness of the throat, and other unpleasant symptoms. Occasionally an allergic response can interfere with breathing and circulation so badly that the sufferer can die. Peanut allergy is a common cause of this severe response.

For a child to develop an allergy to peanuts, she has first to come into contact with traces of peanut. This initial contact sensitises her to peanuts – it sets things up for later allergic responses. Because most allergic children react badly when they are first given peanuts in food, experts assume that they have been sensitised by some earlier, non-food contact.

Pregnancy

It is possible that this contact may take place during pregnancy when a tiny quantity of peanut protein, or related substance, crosses the placenta to the baby. Although there is no firm evidence to support this theory – but because peanut allergy is such a serious problem – the UK government now recommends that some women avoid peanuts while they are pregnant.

You are advised to avoid peanuts if you, the father of your baby or your existing children have an allergic condition. An allergic condition includes:

❏ asthma
❏ eczema
❏ hay fever
❏ any allergic response to foods such as nuts, shellfish or strawberries.

Breastfeeding and peanuts

Breastfeeding is the best way to feed your baby. Your breastmilk will give your baby real protection against many infections and illness. Breastfed babies are less likely than babies fed on artificial baby milks to develop allergic conditions.

There is a small chance that breastfed babies may come into contact with peanuts through their mother's milk. For this reason, the UK government recommends that mothers with a personal or family background of allergic conditions should continue to avoid peanuts while they are breastfeeding.

Avoiding peanuts

Please note – these are guidelines for pregnant and breastfeeding women only. Children with peanut allergy need to be a lot more careful. See your doctor or a dietitian.

❑ Avoid peanut butter and raw peanuts (also called ground nuts or monkey nuts).

❑ Read food labels carefully for mention of 'peanuts' or simply 'nuts' (in particular, cereals, biscuits, cakes and muesli – but also some ice creams and salad dressings).

❑ Ask your supermarket for a list of peanut-free products.

❑ Ask in restaurants if the dish of your choice contains peanuts (if in doubt, choose a simple meal in which the ingredients are obvious).

❑ Don't worry about avoiding 'refined peanut oil' – there is no proof that this causes an allergy.

Key points

❏ Your body is designed to nurture your baby, both before and after her birth. If you cannot eat a healthy diet for some reason, your body's stores of nutrients will be used to meet your baby's needs. If your diet has been poor for some time, you may need a multivitamin and mineral supplement. Choose one without vitamin A.

❏ So-called 'junk' food can be part of a balanced diet – so long as foods such as pizza are combined with plenty of fruit and vegetables.

❏ Dental care is important during pregnancy, and treatment is free from NHS dentists. Mercury fillings are not recommended during pregnancy.

❏ During pregnancy the iron in your blood becomes more diluted. This does not mean that you automatically need iron tablets. However, some women (very young women, women with very heavy periods) do become genuinely anaemic during pregnancy and need treatment.

❏ Continue to take care with food safety when eating out or travelling abroad. Go to popular eating places with good, clean facilities, and choose simple, freshly prepared and well-cooked meals.

❑ Organic foods are good for everybody – but their present high cost and poor supply are major drawbacks for many people.

❑ Avoid peanuts during pregnancy and breastfeeding if you, your baby's father, or your existing children have an allergic condition.

8

After the birth

It may be hard finding the words to describe how you feel now that your baby is born. Joyful – relieved – delighted – amazed – proud. Yes – feel proud of yourself! You have done something wonderful and special – so enjoy the congratulations and the good wishes. You deserve it all!

But for many women this can be a time of mixed emotions. Some women may find their happiness tinged with regret and sadness, because things have not gone as they hoped. Many new mothers feel overwhelmed by the responsibility of caring for their new baby.

As well as dealing with this mix of emotions, you are also faced with the physical effects of giving birth – bruising, soreness, backache, maybe problems with bladder or bowels. Many women simply feel very, very tired, but find they cannot rest because their babies (or other family members) seem to need them continually.

It may seem that everybody's attention is now on your

baby. You may not want it to be any other way – but it can make it harder to find time to think about your own needs and to look after yourself.

You and your midwife

Many of the things that happen to your body – and your mind – after the birth of your baby will get better as time passes. Some things, however, need expert advice or medical treatment.

Don't suffer in silence! If anything about your health bothers you, either in hospital or at home – ask your midwife. She is the expert in the care of mothers and small babies. Along with your GP, your midwife is there to advise and care for you in the early days as you recover from childbirth and get to know your baby.

After the first week or two, your health visitor will be on hand to provide information and support for you and your growing baby.

Easy to forget!

'Packets of crisps and coffee – that's all I had time for! But I felt awful – bloated and cross.'

In the middle of all the excitement and hard work of looking after your baby, it is very easy to forget the importance of eating a healthy diet. But, just as your baby depended on you for nourishment during pregnancy, she depends on you now for food and love, comfort and security. Whether you are breastfeeding or not, your health and energy and your baby's wellbeing are closely connected. It may seem difficult to find the time to eat well, but you owe it to your baby to look after yourself!

In this chapter we talk about the realities of healthy eating after the birth of your baby. We also talk about weight changes. Some women are worried about extra weight gained during pregnancy – others are less concerned. We talk about when – and how – it is safe to start trying to lose weight following the birth of your baby.

The early days

'Breakfast in hospital was marvellous and served to you in bed. It was luxurious just lying there and letting people look after you!'

Many women want just two things after their baby is born: a cup of tea or other refreshing drink, and a good sleep with their baby close by. Later on, you may start to feel very hungry – especially if you have not been able to eat during labour. If you are at home, eat whatever you like and enjoy it! If you are in hospital and a meal is not due, things may be more difficult. The staff on most postnatal wards should be able to give you some toast, breakfast cereal or a cold snack. You may also like to make sure you have a supply of food with you, perhaps in a small cool box: some bananas, apples, crackers and cheese, a sachet of instant soup mix and a bread roll, some nuts and raisins, digestive biscuits, oat and syrup flapjack – whatever!

The food supplied by hospitals varies a lot. Many women are very happy with the meals they are given, but some feel that the portions are inadequate. Other women find that there are not enough vegetables and fruit, and other sources of fibre. Ask your visitors to keep you supplied with small, easily eaten fruit – bananas, satsumas, apricots, apples.

Tell the staff on the postnatal ward if you need special food, such as diabetic, vegetarian, halal or kosher. Some women prefer to ask their relatives to bring food into hospital for them to eat, especially if they are only staying for a short time. The staff on postnatal wards are used to this happening.

Don't forget to drink!

'I longed for a pint-mug of tea . . .'

Hospital wards can be very warm places – and breastfeeding is thirsty work! Drink as much water as you can – aiming for at least two and a half jugs in 24 hours. You could take some low-sugar fruit squash into hospital with you, or some bottles of fizzy water.

Drinking plenty is one of the best ways of easing

constipation and preventing infections in your urine. You may not feel like walking frequently to the toilet, but doing so will help your blood circulation.

If you have had a caesarean section

It takes a bit longer to start eating again after a caesarean section. This is because any big abdominal operation (like a caesarean section) interferes temporarily with the working of your bowels. It may take 2–3 days for your gut to move freely again. If you eat too much before this happens, you may be sick.

Before you have your operation, an intravenous infusion (IVI) will be started. An IVI is the giving of fluid directly into one of your veins, through a fine, flexible needle and tube. A long and difficult labour without drinking leaves you dry and weak. More fluid and blood is lost during an operation. An IVI keeps your body supplied with fluid, and makes it easier to give a blood transfusion if this is required.

Your IVI will continue to give you fluid after your operation. It will be painlessly removed when your midwife feels that you are drinking enough water. This is generally possible within 24 hours of the birth of your baby by caesarean section – but may sometimes take longer.

Once you are drinking water, you may be offered a 'light diet' – which means easily digested foods. Some surgeons prefer even this to wait until your bowels are fully working. Your midwife or doctor may ask you if you have 'passed wind'. This is a sign that your bowels are once again moving. Alternatively, your midwife or doctor may use a stethoscope to listen, through your tummy, for the small noises made when bowels are working properly. Once your bowels are back to normal (generally within three days), you should return to eating a normal, balanced diet.

Trapped wind

Many women who have had their babies by caesarean section are troubled by trapped wind, caused by sluggish bowels in the first two days. This can be very painful. Movement often helps. If you are still in bed, ask your midwife to help you sit up and support you as you carefully bend forwards from the waist a few times. If you can get out of bed, ask somebody to steady you as you walk around a little. Your midwife will give you painkillers and other suitable drugs, either in a medicine or, later, in a suppository (a small capsule to insert into your back passage). These drugs will not harm your breastfeeding baby.

A caesarean section is a major operation, from which your body takes at least six weeks to recover. Look after yourself. Before you leave hospital, you may like to ask your midwife to explain exactly why your caesarean section was necessary, rather than worry about this later at home. At home, you will need extra household help for several weeks while you concentrate on your baby.

Anaemia

Whether or not you were told you were anaemic during pregnancy, it is a good idea to make sure you are eating enough foods rich in iron. You may be offered a blood test to check your haemoglobin, when your baby is 3–5 days old. By this time your blood has returned to its non-pregnant state and is no longer diluted by the extra fluid carried during pregnancy.

❑ Include one item one of iron-rich food in every meal. Your body can only absorb a limited amount of iron – so large portions are not necessary. Look again at the list in Chapter 2.

❑ You can eat liver again now! Liver is rich in iron, full of vitamins and protein, and low in fat.

❑ Try this easy vegan recipe for extra iron, zinc and calcium: Blend cooked black-eyed beans with plenty of tahini, tomato paste and crushed garlic to taste. Eat on toast, in sandwiches, or add to vegetable soup.

Don't forget that your body needs vitamin C to absorb the iron from non-meat sources of iron. Try fortified breakfast cereal with grapefruit juice, baked beans on wholemeal toast with spring onions, or cashew nuts with rice and peppers.

Going to the toilet

It may be 2–3 days before your bowels open. This is normal; you probably emptied your bowels at the start of labour, and then had very little to eat for 12–24 hours. If you have stitches in your perineum or around your back passage, you may feel very anxious about going to the toilet. (The perineum is the area between the opening to your vagina and your back passage.) Try not to worry. Your stitches are very secure. They will not tear when your bowels open because the whole area is very stretchy.

❏ Avoid getting constipated by drinking plenty of water and increasing the amount of roughage in your diet. Take with you into hospital a small packet of high-fibre breakfast cereal and some dried fruit such as figs, prunes or apricots.

❏ If you have a lot of stitches your midwife may offer you a drug to add bulk to your faeces. Passing a large, soft motion will be more comfortable than a small, hard one.

❏ If you are troubled by haemorrhoids, ask your midwife for some ointment to soothe and reduce them.

❏ When you go to the toilet, try to relax and breathe slowly. Some women find it helps to hold a clean sanitary towel or pad of tissue against their perineum as their bowels open.

At home with your baby

'My sister came to stay because my husband was away. She really knew how to look after me – went out to buy watercress to boost my iron, made me lots of milky drinks . . . '

Every new mother needs a quiet time at home with her new baby – time to get to know her, learn to feed and care for her, and introduce her to other members of the family. You need time, too, to take care of yourself – to eat, rest, wash and think. This time should be free of worries about cooking, shopping and cleaning. It should, ideally, be a special time when you are fed and cared for – so that you, in turn, can care for your baby. For some women this special time will last only a few days, for others it may be several weeks.

You can prepare for this time during pregnancy:

❏   Think about who will be with you at home after your baby is born. It may be your partner, a close friend, your mother or another female relative. Do not expect this person to be and do all things – you may need help from a number of people!

❏   Accept gladly any offers of help. Other people may not do things exactly your way – but anything that gives you time to look after yourself and your baby will help.

❏   Women in some circumstances may be able to get extra help, either from social services or a charity.

This help may be available if, for example, you are unsupported by a partner, have a disability or long-term illness, are expecting more than one baby, or have other young children with special needs. Talk with your midwife, GP or social worker.

❑ Alternatively, you may be able to put some money aside during pregnancy to pay for a few hours' household help once your baby is born.

❑ Stock up gradually on convenience foods – tinned soup, fish, beans, dried fruit, pasta, long-life milk and cheese, frozen fish and meat. Find out in advance if local shops or take-away restaurants deliver goods and meals.

Gifts of food

'A friend from work brought me meals for the freezer. I was really spoilt.'

Think about how other people can help you. In many parts of the world there is a strong tradition of bringing gifts of food to new mothers. Food may not be so beautiful as a bunch of flowers from a shop – but it is much more useful (and often cheaper). Could you ask visiting family and friends to bring food? Maybe a casserole ready to heat up, a pie to put in the oven, prepared vegetables or salad to keep in the fridge, a cake, fresh bread or fruit?

Alternatively, could you ask visitors to cook a simple meal? Perhaps prepare a baked potato and filling, fix sardines on toast, make macaroni cheese, wash salad ingredients? (Or just do the washing-up!)

A few women feel ready to go out shopping within a few days of giving birth – but most feel that it is better to stay at home for at least a week. Do you have a neighbour who can collect some things for you while she is doing her own food shopping? Could you ask a friend to pick up the occasional take-away meal for you?

Remember that people really want to help when there is a new baby – but often do not know what to do for the best.

Moving on

As soon as your baby is born, your body begins to get back to normal. Levels of progesterone – one of the hormones of pregnancy – fall rapidly when the placenta leaves your body. Your breasts start to make milk (whether or not you choose to breastfeed). Smooth muscle tone throughout your body quickly improves, and heartburn and constipation get better within days.

You will probably find that you pass large amounts of urine in the first 2–3 days after the birth of your baby. This is the extra fluid carried in pregnancy. Your circulation and breathing will now start getting back to normal.

Your uterus, which weighed about 1kg (2.2lb) at the end of pregnancy, gets rapidly smaller. The muscular walls contract, and then start getting thinner. By the time your baby is six weeks old, your uterus is almost back to its pre-pregnant weight of 50g (2oz).

Your abdominal muscles regain their tone within a couple of months – after being stretched to twice their length late in pregnancy. Regular, gentle exercise that you enjoy will help build up the strength of these muscles. Your midwife, or a hospital physiotherapist, should tell you about suitable exercises for the early weeks. Make sure you know how to exercise your pelvic floor muscles.

Weight changes after pregnancy

'I felt the weight drop off me when my son was born – but I still couldn't get into my favourite clothes at first. I was so disappointed.'

Immediately following childbirth most women still weigh more than they did before they got pregnant. Many women accept this extra 'cuddliness' as part of being a mother. Some, for the first time in their lives, welcome the chance to be more relaxed about the size and shape of their bodies.

Other women are disturbed about being larger than they think they should be. Getting back to their normal weight is extremely important to them. A few women will be so worried that they start to try to lose weight in an unsafe way, and may even develop an eating disorder (such as anorexia or bulimia) as they try to take control of their situation. Talk things over with your health visitor or GP if you feel that worries about what you are eating are taking over your life.

You may like to read again the short section in Chapter 5 about working out your Body Mass Index (BMI). Your

BMI is an objective measure of how overweight (or underweight) you really are. You may find that you are not so overweight as you think!

Take care!

It is not a good idea for any new mother – breast-feeding or not – to try to lose weight too quickly. Aiming to lose more than 0.5kg (1lb) a week will leave you tired, miserable and open to infection and illness. Likewise, restricting what you eat before breastfeeding has really got going (6–8 weeks) may reduce your supply of milk. In fact, research has shown that regularly eating less than 1,800kcals a day at any time while breastfeeding is likely to reduce the quality and quantity of the breastmilk you produce.

You will naturally lose some weight after your baby is born. Why not wait until this natural weight loss has stopped before cutting down on what you eat? Many breastfeeding mothers prefer to wait until their baby starts taking some solid food (at around six months). In the meantime, paying attention to your posture and doing any kind of enjoyable exercise will help tone and strengthen your body.

Not eating enough?

'I was thinner within six weeks of having my baby than I was before I got pregnant. I was like a bean-pole.'

Looking after a young baby is very hard work. Many women feel, at times, simply too tired and too stressed to eat. Alone at home with your baby, it may not always seem worth the effort of preparing a 'proper meal' for just one person. Some women worry about losing too much weight.

❑ Keep in mind the basic healthy eating plan – eating the correct balance of food is as important now as it ever has been.

❑ If the idea of preparing meals is too much, think instead about eating a series of healthy snacks throughout the day. Look again at the list of nutritious, no-cook snacks in Chapter 4.

❑ Prepare snacks for the day ahead when you have time – get a tin of baked beans out of the cupboard, scrub a large potato and put it in the oven to cook slowly, chop salad ingredients, hard-boil an egg, make some tuna sandwiches, put ready a packet of high-fibre breakfast cereal.

❑ Sleep – or at least sit with your feet up and read a magazine – when your baby is asleep.

Natural weight changes

'I didn't diet or anything . . . I was breastfeeding
him and, after a few months, the weight just melted
off. I got quite worried!'

We do not know for sure what happens naturally to a
woman's weight after her baby is born. Research into
weight loss after childbirth is hard because very few
women in Western society leave things completely to
nature.

This is what we know so far. The most rapid weight
loss occurs in the first three days as the body loses the
extra fluid that it carried during pregnancy. Natural
weight loss after this is much slower, regardless of feeding
method. Research indicates that it is unrealistic for a
mother to expect her weight to return to normal for at
least six months after having her baby. Some experts feel
that it may take nearly a year.

Some women feel that breastfeeding helps them to lose
weight. Others find that their appetite increases dramatically
while breastfeeding and so their weight stays the same.
There is, however, evidence that breastfeeding women
find it easier to lose fat from around their hips and thighs
than mothers using artificial baby milks.

Breastfeeding women tend to lose most weight when:

❑   they feed their babies frequently during the first three
    months, and do not use any artificial baby milk

❑ they continue to breastfeed for longer than six months – as nature intends.

Women do not often become overweight because of pregnancy. Men – and women who do not have children – also tend to get larger as the years go by. Lack of exercise and unhealthy eating patterns are more likely to make us overweight than having babies.

Exercise – it's worth the effort!

'I didn't really do any real exercise until he was over a year old – I just didn't have time. Then a friend took me swimming – and it made me feel so good – it was unbelievable! I won't wait so long next time.'

Before you start worrying about cutting back on what you eat, think about the benefits of exercise. Regular exercise:

❑ helps you lose weight
❑ tones and strengthens your muscles
❑ makes you feel good, mentally as well as physically.

Finding the time – and energy – to exercise may seem very hard. But it really is worth it! When you exercise, even for a short time, chemicals released in your body actually make you feel more energetic and more positive about life in general.

You may feel that your baby needs you all the time and you cannot leave her with anybody else. So what about taking her along with you? Many community and leisure centres run exercise classes for new mothers, with babies cared for close by. Ask your health visitor what is available in your area, and look for information on noticeboards in your health centre and library. Swimming, too, is very good exercise. Some swimming pools have crèches for older babies – or could you take a friend along to share the babycare?

At home, try running upstairs each time you need to go up without your baby. What about skipping like you did at school – or using a hula-hoop? Neither activity takes up much room or needs special preparation. Put the radio on and skip or twirl for the duration of a song. Energetic dancing is good exercise, too. Maybe take a long route round to the shops, and walk as fast as you can with your pram or buggy. Think about carrying your baby in a sling or back-pack – the weight of your baby will give you more exercise. Have a look at the exercise videos in your local library. Could you share one with a friend at home?

Remember that exercise taken little and often is better than one long session, especially after having a baby. Start exercising very gently, and build up gradually. Many women prefer to wait until after their GP check-up at six weeks.

The secret of successful weight loss

Forget the idea of making drastic, short-term changes to your diet – and then returning to your normal foods! The best – and most lasting – way to lose weight is to alter the balance of foods you eat and, at the same time, change the way you feel about food so that these alterations become natural to you.

The best foods to avoid are the fatty foods, because fat gives us twice as much energy as the same weight of protein or carbohydrate. Fill up instead on vegetables, fruit and reasonably large quantities of starchy carbohydrate foods like breakfast cereals, bread, pasta and potatoes. This means that you will feel full, without eating so many calories. (Remember that brown, wholemeal cereals and pasta are more filling than white.)

Start telling yourself how much you now dislike fatty foods. Think about the fat in pies, salami and bacon – or the fat that foods like chips and fried bread soak up during cooking. Imagine that fat as a greasy lump, and think about it going straight to your hips or tummy – or whatever part of your body where you want to lose weight.

Read the labels on food. Five grams of fat is about the weight of one those small, wrapped rectangles of butter used in cafes. Imagine the fat in these foods as blobs of oily butter in your body:

❏ a small packet of crisps – 2 blobs (9g fat)
❏ one serving of chips – 3 blobs (17g)

- [ ] an individual pork pie – 6 blobs (30g)
- [ ] one samosa – 5 blobs (26g)
- [ ] a small bar of chocolate – 3 blobs (15g).

Cutting down on fats

Use skimmed milk (less than 1g fat in one pint) or semi-skimmed milk (9g) instead of whole milk (22g fat!). Skimmed milk gives you the same amount of protein and calcium – but far fewer calories. If you find skimmed milk thin at first (especially if you are breastfeeding), whisk an extra teaspoon of skimmed milk powder into a glass of skimmed milk.

White fish and tuna in brine are the animal protein foods lowest in fat. Otherwise, choose low-fat meat such as ham, chicken and turkey. Take the skin off poultry. (Most of the fat on poultry meat is just under the skin and will be removed at the same time.) Choose lean cuts of meat. These are more expensive than fatty cuts – but you don't need such big servings. Cut off any visible fat.

Casserole or stew tougher cuts of meat – but spoon off the fat from the top of the liquid before serving. Leave cooked mince, curries and gravy to stand for a few moments – then drain or spoon away the excess fat that rises to the surface. Grill rather than fry food. Fish can also be steamed or baked.

Choose an unsaturated oil such as sunflower, soya, corn, rapeseed or olive oil for cooking – and use as little as possible. Avoid saturated fats such as lard and butter.

Instead of using margarine or butter on bread, try thinly spread low-calorie mayonnaise, fromage frais or salad cream. Moist sandwich fillings do not really need any spread at all.

Avoid pastry items such as pork pies, sausage rolls and individual meat pies. If you have chips (as a special treat!), cut them straight and thick – less surface area to absorb fat. Remember that a serving of roast potatoes contains 9g fat, compared with 0.2g fat in a portion of boiled potatoes.

Be a label watcher! Sausages, for example, can vary from being 33% fat to less than 10%. A small pot of full-fat yoghurt contains 3.5g fat, while a low-fat one has just 1g. A 50g (2oz) chunk of Cheddar cheese contains 19g fat, compared with 8.4g in a low-fat variety – or 2.1g in cottage cheese.

Watch the sugar too!

Sugar is another source of 'empty calories'. Not only does sugar not provide any vitamins and minerals, but it actually drains nutrients from your body as it is digested. This is even more important when you are limiting what you eat in order to lose weight.

Hidden sugars

Many processed foods have an alarming amount of added sugar:

- serving of tomato ketchup: 1 teaspoon of sugar
- glass of diluted orange squash: 2.5 teaspoons
- small pot of fruit yoghurt: 4 teaspoons
- can of soft drink: 7 teaspoons
- small chocolate bar: 7.5 teaspoons

Tips for cutting down on sugar

- Try to reduce, or stop taking, sugar in tea and coffee. It may taste awful for about a week – then you begin to realise how good the drink is without sweetness!
- Choose low-calorie soft drinks – they contain artificial sweeteners in place of sugar.
- Choose breakfast cereals with 'no added sugar'.
- Sugar in processed foods may be hidden under different names – check the label carefully for 'dextrose', 'glucose', 'fructose' and 'maltose' as well as 'sugar'. Buy tinned fruit preserved in natural juice rather than syrup.
- Halve the sugar in recipes when baking at home – it works for most things except meringues

and jam. (Bake low-sugar, low-fat wholemeal scones or biscuits, packed with dried fruit, for healthy snacks.)

❑ Use artificial sweeteners if you have a very sweet tooth. Try aspartame, saccharin and ace-suffame K in place of sugar in drinks, on cereals or to sweeten sour fruit. There is no evidence that the small amounts needed are harmful during pregnancy or breastfeeding.

Try this . . .

❑ Don't go shopping when you are hungry – you'll come back with completely different foods from those you planned to buy!

❑ Don't let yourself get too hungry – or you'll be tempted to reach for cakes and biscuits. Keep handy a supply of healthy snacks – fruit that you enjoy, washed and chopped vegetables, breadsticks and crispbreads (no spread!).

❑ Don't forget to drink plenty of water or other low-calorie drinks. A hot drink often seems to fill you up if you begin to feel hungry between meals. Try a mug of yeast or beef extract mixed with hot water, a low-calorie soup mix or fruit tea.

More help needed?

'I just didn't have the willpower! Then my sister and I decided we'd lose weight together. Now we phone each other if we feel tempted.'

If, after trying some of these ideas, you still feel very worried about your weight, talk things over with your GP. She will make sure that there is no hidden medical reason for your weight, and may then suggest that you take advice from a state registered dietitian. You do not have to pay to see a dietitian; your GP will make the necessary arrangements.

Alternatively, many women find it very useful to join an organisation such as Weight Watchers. Weight Watchers give support and lots of encouragement to women wanting to reduce their weight. They also have programmes tailored to individual needs – breastfeeding mothers, for example. You will have to pay to join and to attend regular meetings. Look in your phone book for a local contact.

Don't rush into dieting after your baby is born – it may be best to wait until you have stopped losing weight naturally. In the meantime, aim to get some regular exercise. Later, if you feel you still need to lose weight, cut right back on fats – and keep to the basic plan for healthy eating.

Key points

❑ Life with a new baby is very busy, but try to remember the importance of a balanced diet. You owe it to yourself and your baby!

❑ Relieve constipation by drinking plenty of water, and increasing the amount of roughage in your diet. Prevent anaemia by including one iron-rich food and a source of vitamin C in every meal.

❑ Try to prepare in advance for the early days at home with your new baby. Make sure you have plenty of practical help, especially with shopping and food preparation.

❑ Natural weight loss after childbirth can be slow. It may take nearly a year to return naturally to your pre-pregnant weight. If you want to lose weight more quickly cut down on all fatty foods and fill up with vegetables, fruit, and reasonable quantities of starchy carbohydrates. It is not good to try to lose more than 0.5kg (1lb) a week.

❑ When you feel ready, try to take some regular exercise. Start gently, and remember that exercise taken little and often is better than one long session. Don't forget your pelvic floor exercises!

❑ Breastfeeding helps some women to lose weight, especially if you feed on demand, and continue to feed for longer than six months. Your milk supply may be affected if you try to lose weight too early (before 6–8 weeks) or too quickly (by eating less than 1,800 calories a day. It may be best to wait until you baby starts taking solid food before cutting down on what you eat.

9

Breastfeeding

'Breastfeeding was so important to me. I was giving my baby everything she needed and it gave me a chance to sit and just be with her.'

In some ways, this should be the first rather than the last chapter in this book – because breastfeeding gives your baby the very best start in life. Breastmilk will give your baby health benefits that will stay with her throughout her life, until she has her own babies – and beyond.

Human breastmilk is designed exclusively for human babies. It is the ultimate convenience food. Throughout this book, we've used the image of a plate of food to help balance our meals and make sure we have all the protein, energy, water, vitamins and minerals that we need. But there is no need for the plate plan with breastmilk! All the nutrients needed by your baby for the first half of her first year are there, clean, fresh, ready made, ready mixed – and ready heated.

Getting ready for breastfeeding

Your body starts preparing for breastfeeding right at the beginning of pregnancy. Your breasts start growing even before your baby starts moving. Your body lays down stores of energy and other nutrients to help make milk. However early your baby is born, there is colostrum (special concentrated breastmilk for new babies) waiting for her in your breasts.

As soon as your baby and her placenta leave your body, pregnancy hormones fall – and breastfeeding hormones rise. Within 2-3 days, your breasts are making mature milk. This will happen automatically – whether or not you plan to breastfeed. Each time your baby suckles, levels of breastfeeding hormones rise – and more milk is made. The more your baby suckles, the more milk you will produce.

If you decide not to breastfeed, the preparations made by your body for breastfeeding are soon reversed. It may be hard to start breastfeeding later. If you are undecided about how to feed your baby, it is best to try breastfeeding and see how you get on. Whatever you decide to do later, your baby will have had some colostrum. Colostrum is rich in protein and antibodies which will help protect your baby from infections.

In this chapter we talk about looking after yourself while you are breastfeeding. We also answer some of the questions that women ask about how what they eat may affect their breastfeeding baby.

Making plenty of milk

Breastfeeding is a natural part of a busy life. All over the world women produce plenty of milk for their babies while working long and hard.

Lactation (making breastmilk) is a very efficient process. During lactation your metabolism slows slightly to conserve energy, and your body uses food more efficiently. Furthermore, there is rarely any waste; you make just enough milk to suit your baby.

Your supply of breastmilk depends on the needs of your baby. As she grows and needs more, so you produce more. The important thing is to feed her 'on demand' (when she wants to be fed) – and to make sure that she is well 'attached' (or 'positioned') at your breast.

Being well attached means that she has a wide mouthful of breast, including your nipple and some of your areola (the darker skin surrounding the nipple). Feeding like this will not hurt you. A baby who is well attached feeds calmly, and stops feeding naturally when she has had enough.

You do not need to eat enormous quantities of special foods in order to breastfeed – but you do need some extra calories. If a breastfeeding mother cannot eat well (because of illness, maybe, or extreme poverty) she will continue to make breastmilk, but her energy stores will soon be used up. She will feel tired and miserable, and her natural defences against infection will be reduced. Her own health will suffer, even though her baby may grow.

How much extra?

'All my meals were cold by the time I got them but I was so hungry I didn't care. I just ate everything to build up my milk supply for the twins.'

Experts have worked out that breastfeeding women need, on average, an extra 500 calories a day when they are exclusively breastfeeding for several months. The exact amount will vary as time goes by. Women with good fat stores who are less active may need less than this.

As during pregnancy, you don't need to worry about working out how much food to eat. Your appetite will be a good guide – so don't be surprised if you feel very hungry at times. Many women settle into a routine of four meals a day, plenty of drinks, and a snack in the middle of the night.

If this sort of eating pattern works for you, don't worry that this will be too much food and you will never lose weight. Research shows that most women do return eventually to their normal weight, although it may take up to a year for this to happen naturally.

Make sure you drink enough

'I was thirsty as soon as the baby went to the breast. I had to make a point of having a large glass of water beside me every time I fed.'

Many women find that they get very thirsty, especially during the early weeks of breastfeeding. This is not surprising when you consider how much milk you are making.

Don't ignore your thirst! Prepare a jug of low-sugar squash or keep a glass by the tap and drink whenever you feel thirsty. The surge of oxytocin during let-down often makes women feel acutely thirsty. Pour yourself a drink before you sit down to feed. You will probably find you get thirsty during the night as well. Keep a bottle of water or flask of milk in the bedroom ready for night feeds.

There is no need to drink if you are not thirsty. Forcing yourself to drink large quantities of water when you are not thirsty may temporarily reduce your milk supply.

Mixed feeding?

If you are giving your baby just the occasional bottle of artificial baby milk, your needs will probably be much the same as when you are fully breastfeeding. If you are regularly using artificial baby milk as well as breastfeeding, you will probably not have to eat so much as you will be making less breastmilk.

The breastfeeding hormones

❑ Prolactin is the production hormone. The more your baby feeds, well attached to your breast, the more milk you produce.

❑ Oxytocin is the delivery hormone. After your baby has been feeding for a few moments on your thirst-quenching 'foremilk', the sensation of her mouth on your breast stimulates the 'let-down' reflex, when for a few seconds oxytocin surges through your breast causing the tiny muscles surrounding your milk cells to tighten. The rich, nutritious 'hindmilk' is thus released to flow down to your baby.

❑ The action of both these hormones depends on your baby being well attached to your breast.

Healthy 500 for breastfeeding
(how 500 calories look)

Each of these small meals provides all the extra energy, protein and almost all of the vitamins needed while you are breastfeeding. The first seven meals contain at least one-fifth of your total daily calcium requirement, and the remaining two provide at least one-sixth.

- ❑ 3 tablespoons of wheatflakes, 2 tablespoons of rolled oats, a tablespoon each of raisins and sesame seeds, quarter of a pint of semi-skimmed milk, and a large orange (or 7oz glass of orange juice)
- ❑ 2 heaped teaspoons of malted chocolate drink powder mixed into a half-pint mug of hot, semi-skimmed milk; a poached egg and 2 tablespoons of spinach; 2 slices of wholemeal bread with a scraping of soft margarine and yeast extract
- ❑ a strawberry milkshake made with one-third of a pint of semi-skimmed milk, a heaped table-spoon of fresh strawberries, a teaspoon of sugar and a large scoop of ice cream; a third of a pint of lentil soup with a slice of wholemeal bread (no butter)
- ❑ 2 slices of wholemeal bread spread with soya margarine; a matchbox-sized chunk of low-fat Cheddar cheese, with tomato and lettuce; followed by a banana

- 6-inch piece of french bread with 3 teaspoons of low-calorie mayonnaise, 2 slices of lean ham, quarter of a bunch of watercress (or mustard-and-cress) and some chinese leaves
- an individual portion of frozen lasagne; 2 florets of steamed or boiled broccoli; followed by a baked apple with a tablespoon of sultanas and a teaspoon of sugar
- 3 fried, low-fat sausages; 3 medium boiled potatoes (no butter!) and cabbage (or spring greens); stewed fruit and 3 tablespoons of custard made with skimmed milk
- a large baked potato and a teaspoon of sunflower margarine; half a large tin of baked beans; a large green salad
- mackerel paté (made from half a medium-sized smoked mackerel fillet, mashed with a heaped tablespoon of low-fat soft cheese, ground pepper and lemon juice); 3 Ryvita crispbread; and a pepper and sweetcorn salad.

Special needs

'My baby just got bigger and bigger! I started him on solids – but he was still taking a lot of breastmilk. I was getting thinner, my hair went straight and my nails started splitting. To start with, I was eating quite well but I think I forgot . . . it was easier to see what he wanted instead of what I wanted. I'm trying to think more about my food now.'

Your milk will give your baby all the vitamins and minerals she needs, but this may sometimes be at the expense of your reserves. Thinking carefully about what you eat will make sure that your own nutrient levels remain good.

Vegan diets

Vitamin B_{12} is needed for the growth of cells – so your growing baby needs plenty. Vitamin B_{12} is found in meat, fish, eggs, milk, cheese and yoghurt. If you eat any of these foods, you are probably getting enough vitamin B_{12}.

If you do not eat any animal products at all, you may not be getting enough vitamin B_{12}. Vitamin B_{12} is added to fortified foods such as yeast extracts, some margarines, soya milk and soya 'meat' – but you should check the labels carefully. The B group of vitamins are not stored in our bodies, so new supplies are needed each day. You need 2μg (2mcg or 2 microgrammes) vitamin B_{12} a day while breastfeeding. You may feel safer taking a supplement.

Vitamins A and C, and the B group

Vitamin C is another vitamin that needs to be eaten each day. Five portions of vegetables and fruit will probably give you enough vitamin C for breastfeeding. Just one more serving will help provide the extra vitamin A and B group vitamins also needed while breastfeeding. Take another look at Chapter 1 for ideas.

Healthy bones

When you are breastfeeding, your need for calcium and zinc is almost double that of pregnancy. This is because your baby is growing very fast and, at the same time, her bones are hardening. She needs plenty of calcium for this to happen well.

If you like milk, now is the time to drink plenty! Milk is a good source of protein, calcium, zinc, vitamin B_2 and vitamin B_{12}. Drink it cold from the fridge, or in milk shakes. Try whisking in a mashed banana or raspberries – or make lassi by mixing yoghurt with milk and adding a pinch of salt or sugar. A hot milky drink at night can be very comforting – and don't forget milk puddings, custards and sauces. Remember that skimmed and semi-skimmed milk contain the same nutrients as whole milk – but much less fat.

However, you do not need to drink milk to make milk. The box on page 190 shows non-milk foods rich in calcium. If you feel that you can eat the equivalent of 1⅔ pint of milk in these foods a day, your calcium requirement will probably be met. Otherwise, you may like to think about taking a calcium supplement while you are breastfeeding.

Choose a supplement containing around 1,000mg calcium and 10µg (10mcg or 10 microgrammes) vitamin D. You could ask your doctor for a prescription, or ask for tablets yourself from a chemist's shop. Ask the pharmacist for advice before buying.

You will also need extra calcium if you are still growing yourself while you are breastfeeding (if you are aged 18 years or less). Again, a supplement may be a good idea.

Zinc is found in a wide variety of foods, especially the high-protein foods. Look again at the list in Chapter 2. Aim to add an extra portion of meat, cheese or eggs to your diet, plus some wholemeal bread, pasta or breakfast cereal. Wholegrain products are good sources, too, of a mineral called selenium. Selenium is an important antioxidant (see Chapter 2). It is also needed for healthy bones. Selenium is found in fish, cheese and lentils.

Breastfeeding and your bones

Calcium is an important part of the structure of your bones. While you are breastfeeding, calcium is gradually released from your bones. This is normal and, for most women, causes no problems. The calcium released is probably used to make breastmilk. The speed of this release varies a lot from woman to woman. In general, the more milk you produce for your baby, the greater the release of calcium from your bones.

This calcium loss from your bones is only temporary. Your bones start getting back to normal as soon as your baby starts to eat other foods and needs less breastmilk. In fact, research suggests that your bones may be denser (harder) after breastfeeding than they were immediately after the birth of your baby.

Calcium-rich foods

Aim to drink 1⅔ pints of milk a day – or the equivalent in other dairy products or non-milk foods. A matchbox-sized portion of Cheddar cheese and a small pot of yoghurt both contain the same calcium as a third of a pint of milk.

Non-milk calcium foods

These are equivalent to a third of a pint of milk:

- ❏ 2 sardines from a tin of fish in oil
- ❏ one-sixth of a pack of tofu
- ❏ 1 glass (7oz) of calcium enriched soya milk
- ❏ 5 dried figs

These are equivalent to one-sixth of a pint of milk:

- ❏ 3 medium slices of white bread
- ❏ 24 whole almonds
- ❏ 2 tablespoons of cooked spinach
- ❏ 1 tablespoon of sesame seeds or tahini

More than one baby?

Yes – you can make enough milk for more than one baby! Some women may be still breastfeeding an older child, as well as a new baby. Others will give birth to twins, or more. The key – as always – is to feed on demand (remembering that this may take a lot of time in the early weeks), and eat and drink to satisfy your appetite.

You will probably feel constantly hungry as your need for energy, protein, zinc and calcium increase dramatically. All of these nutrients are found in dairy products. If you do not like milk, it may be a good idea to take a calcium supplement. Although there are other food sources of calcium besides milk (see opposite and Chapter 2), it is hard to get enough calcium for double milk production without using dairy products.

The vitamin D question

We need a good supply of vitamin D to absorb calcium from food, and to use this calcium in our bones. If we do not get enough vitamin D, our bones get softer. In adults this is called osteomalacia. In children the condition is called rickets; their soft bones bend as they grow. Some children in the UK have rickets.

We can get vitamin D from oily fish, eggs, margarine and dairy products. Our bodies also make vitamin D – but need the sun to do this. In the UK, the winter sun is not strong enough. During the winter, if we do not eat vitamin D foods, we rely on body stores left over from the summer.

Some people may have low stores of vitamin D (look again at Chapter 2). The government recommend that breastfeeding women take a 10µg (10mcg or 10 micro-grammes) supplement of vitamin D. This is particularly important if:

❑ you rarely expose your skin to the sun in summer, and
❑ you don't like foods rich in vitamin D.

Ask your health visitor about vitamin D supplements.

'Why does my breastfed baby need extra vitamin K?'

Vitamin K is needed to help blood clot and so stop bleeding. A tiny number of babies (around one in every 10,000) are at risk of bleeding because they do not have enough vitamin K. Sometimes this shortage is caused by illness, but often we do not know the cause. Whatever the cause, although bleeding due to a shortage of vitamin K is very rare, it can be fatal.

Doctors recommend that all babies be given extra vitamin K at birth. It can be given either by injection, or in a few drops of medicine. Some parents think that levels are low for a particular reason that we do not yet understand, and choose not to give extra vitamin K.

The vitamin K injection will prevent all bleeding due to low levels of vitamin K. There is, however, a small possibility that there is some link between this injection and some childhood cancers. Although most experts feel that this is unlikely, the possibility cannot be completely ruled out.

If your baby has the vitamin K drops at birth, doctors recommend further doses over the next two months. If she is breastfed, she will probably have another dose when she is a week old, and a further one at about six weeks. Artificial baby milk has extra vitamin K added to it already.

Fatty acids

Your baby's brain continues to grow rapidly after birth. Nutrients called 'long chain fatty acids' play an important part.

There are two ways of getting long chain fatty acids (or 'long chain polyunsaturates', as they are sometimes called). First, they are found in foods such as oily fish, lean meat, liver and egg yolk. Second, our bodies can convert linolenic acid and linoleic acid (the two essential fatty acids – see Chapter 1) into long chain fatty acids. Linolenic acid and linoleic acid are found in nuts and vegetable oils, and in oily fish, eggs and lean meat.

Fatty acids are also stored in body fat. They will be released and used in your breastmilk as you lose weight. The level of fatty acids in your breastmilk will reflect both the quantity of fatty acids in your diet and the breakdown of your fat stores.

Getting help with breastfeeding

It takes 6–8 weeks for breastfeeding to really get going – for mother and baby to learn the technique and your milk supply to be fully in tune with your baby's needs. Learning any new skill while adapting to a new way of life – can be very hard. Loving support and sound information can make all the difference.

❑ Your partner: women are more likely to enjoy breast-feeding if their partners support and understand what they are doing.

❑ Family: your mother and mother-in-law may have a lot of breastfeeding experience – but keep in mind that ideas do change over time, so you may get different advice from different people!

❑ Friends: more and more women are choosing to breastfeed. A group of friends who are happily breastfeeding their babies will give each other wonderful support.

❑ Your midwife and health visitor: although individual experience varies, both will have had special training in advising and helping breastfeeding mothers.

❑ A breastfeeding counsellor or supporter: phone the NCT Breastfeeding Line (0870 444 8708) to reach a local breastfeeding counsellor any day between 8am and 10pm. You do not have to be a member of the NCT to speak with a breastfeeding counsellor. Alternatively, ask your midwife or health visitor about local members of the Breastfeeding Network, La Leche League or Association of Breastfeeding Mothers.

❑ Leaflets: there are many very good leaflets and books dealing with breastfeeding. If this is your first baby, ask your midwife or GP for your free copy of *The Pregnancy Book*. Try www.nctpregnancyandbabycare.com for information on breastfeeding or call 0870 112 1120 or visit www.nctms.co.uk for the leaflets *Breastfeeding, A Good Start* and *Breastfeeding, How to express and store your milk*.

Exercise that you enjoy

It is not a good idea to cut back on what you eat while you are breastfeeding. But, when you feel ready, think about getting some exercise. Little and often is best with a new baby.

❏ Moderate exercise will not affect your milk production – provided you continue to feed your baby whenever she is hungry, eat a balanced diet and drink to quench your thirst.

❏ Some women find that they lose weight too quickly when exercising! Make sure that you do not lose more than 0.5kg (1lb) a week – or 2kg (4lb) a month. You may need to snack between meals to slow your weight loss.

❏ You will feel more comfortable wearing a firm, supporting bra when running and jumping.

❏ Reports that babies may dislike the taste of breastmilk after their mothers have been exercising are probably exaggerated. All over the world, women work long and hard while they are breastfeeding, their babies feeding happily throughout.

Drugs and breastfeeding

Take care!

Aspirin can be very harmful to babies. Do not give her aspirin in any form. Ask your doctor, health visitor or pharmacist to recommend a safe drug to ease pain and fever.

Do not take even aspirin yourself, because traces of it will pass through to your baby in your breastmilk. Look carefully at the packet of any drugs you buy – many treatments for colds and 'flu contain aspirin. Paracetamol is generally a safer alternative – but check first with your pharmacist.

Some laxatives (drugs taken to relieve constipation) can also be harmful to breastfed babies. The type that add bulk, rather than stimulate the bowel, are thought to be safer. (Better still – refer back to Chapter 1 of this book for information about increasing the amount of fibre in your diet, and relieving constipation naturally.)

Most drugs pass through in small quantities to your milk – but only a few are so harmful that you have to stop breastfeeding in order to take them. In most cases, the advantages of breastmilk far outweigh any risk of harm to your baby.

Always tell your doctor, dentist or pharmacist that you are breastfeeding so that they can offer you the safest form of treatment. Very occasionally a woman is told that she has to stop breastfeeding in order to take a certain drug or have a treatment such as radiotherapy or a general anaesthetic. You may have a number of choices.

❑ You could check the information given by your doctor with a pharmacist (pharmacists generally have access to the most up-to-date information on drugs).

❑ You could ask your doctor if it is possible to delay the drug treatment until you have naturally weaned your baby.

❑ You could make plans to stop breastfeeding temporarily – but keep your supply going by regularly expressing your breastmilk. The milk you express is thrown away until it is clear of the drug, and your baby is fed on previously stored breastmilk or artificial baby milk.

❑ You could stop breastfeeding and feed your baby on artificial baby milk. If you do this, it is very important that you guard against engorgement and mastitis by cutting down gradually the number of breastfeeds or (if this is not possible) expressing your breasts as often as it takes to keep them soft and comfortable.

Caffeine

Caffeine in tea, coffee, coca cola and chocolate passes quickly into your breastmilk. Babies are not able to metabolise caffeine well. Too much caffeine may make your baby irritable and wakeful. Most women find that it is best to drink no more than three mugs of coffee (or the equivalent – see Chapter 6), and to spread this intake throughout each day. Smoking increases the effect of caffeine.

Smoking and breastfeeding

Your baby is exposed twice over to the effects of your smoking. First, she breathes in your cigarette smoke – and that of anybody else nearby. This will increase her risk of lung disease and dying from cot death.

Second, the chemicals in cigarette smoke pass quickly from your blood into your milk, and so into your baby. Babies of smokers tend to cry more and have more colic. In addition, smoking more than 20 cigarettes a day may:

❏   reduce your milk supply
❏   interfere with your let–down reflex
❏   cause sickness and vomiting in your baby.

The birth of your baby is a good time to stop smoking – and encourage anybody else who lives with you to do the same. Low-dose nicotine patches may be safe to use while breastfeeding. Ask your pharmacist for up-to-date information. Say that you are breastfeeding. The safety of nicotine chewing gum during breastfeeding has not been proven. Prolactin, the main breastfeeding hormone, has a natural calming effect – feed your baby when she wants to feed to keep your prolactin levels high!

If you really cannot stop smoking:

❑ keep breastfeeding! – it will help protect your baby from infection and illness
❑ eat a balanced diet – plenty of fruit and vegetables, and starchy carbohydrates for energy
❑ cut down the number of cigarettes you smoke – as in pregnancy, the fewer cigarettes you smoke, the less the risk of harm to your baby
❑ smoke low-nicotine cigarettes
❑ smoke just after a breastfeed to reduce the amount of nicotine in your milk
❑ never smoke near to your baby
❑ make sure your baby sleeps in a smoke-free room.

Cannabis

Regular use of cannabis while breastfeeding your baby may be extremely harmful. Research has shown that this drug damages the brain cells of newborn animals. Use of cannabis – and all other street drugs – may affect your ability to care for your baby. Get help now, for the safety of your baby.

Alcohol and breastfeeding

'I used to worry about even a small glass of wine . . . My baby was very tiny and if she slept a lot I worried she was drunk!'

Alcohol passes quickly into your blood and then into your breastmilk. Levels in your milk rise and fall as blood levels rise and fall – alcohol is not stored in the breast. You may also notice a distinct smell to your milk after you have drunk alcohol.

❑ The amount of alcohol in your milk peaks 30–60 minutes after having a drink (60–90 minutes if taken with food).
❑ Levels in your blood and your milk return to normal 2–3 hours after a single glass of wine or

normal-strength beer (the more you drink, the longer it will take).

Heavy drinking while breastfeeding (6 units of alcohol a day) may slow your baby's motor development. (Motor development means her ability to walk, use her hands, and so on.) High levels of alcohol in your milk will make your baby either irritable and wakeful, or very sleepy. She may be too sleepy to feed and so her growth will also be affected. You will not be able to look after her safely if you have been drinking heavily, and she should not sleep in your bed.

The effects of more moderate drinking are not really clear. Alcohol use may temporarily affect prolactin levels. Moderate drinking may also delay your let-down reflex. Your baby has to suckle for longer to get the milk she wants – so feeds take longer.

Occasional drinking or regular light drinking (one or fewer drinks each day) has not been found to be harmful to breastfed babies.

> ## 'I've been told that drinking stout will help my milk supply. Is this true?'
>
> This has not been scientifically proven. But, as with many traditional ideas, there may be a grain of truth somewhere! If you are used to drinking alcohol, a small alcoholic drink may help you to relax and unwind – especially if somebody else brings it to you. A cool drink of beer after a hot and tiring day, a glass of wine, a cup of tea, a small coffee – all help us feel cared for and so make it a little easier for us to care for others.

Colic

Colic is a sort of abdominal (tummy) pain suffered by some babies from a few weeks of age until they are 3–4 months old. A baby with colic often cries even when she is well fed, warm and dry, and being held by her mother. She may cry for several hours at almost the same time of day each day.

Nobody knows for sure what causes colic in babies. Some people think that babies suffer colic because their digestive systems are not quite ready to cope with large quantities of lactose (milk sugar). If you think your baby has colic, ask your doctor to check her over. There may be another cause for her crying.

Looking after a baby with colic is very difficult. It is not your fault that your baby has colic. Both bottle-fed and breastfed babies can get colic (but it is often easier to comfort your baby if you are breastfeeding).

Try to get help. A friend may be able to help you comfort your baby while she is crying – or perhaps care for your other children. Your health visitor will give you support and advice. Other mothers will understand what you are going through, and may have good ideas for easing colic. A breastfeeding counsellor or supporter may be able to suggest different breastfeeding techniques.

If you are alone and getting desperate, put your crying baby gently down in her cot, and phone Serene/CRY-SIS, a charity that supports and advises the parents of crying babies: 020 7404 5011 (8am–11pm, 7 days a week).

'Should I change my diet?'

'I was fixated about what I ate – convinced that everything had a direct effect on my baby's colic. It was so bad I stopped orange juice, apples and almost every other fruit and vegetable!'

Many women feel that colic is caused by certain foods that they eat. This may be true but there has not been any large-scale research to prove or disprove this. There is no need to avoid spicy foods or garlic, oranges, onions or cabbage – or any other foods – unless these are upsetting your own digestion. (But don't forget that smoking, and too much caffeine, seems to be linked to colic in some breastfed babies.)

Some experts feel that very occasionally colic may be caused by a baby's reaction to cow's milk protein in her mother's diet. If you have tried everything else, you may like to cut out all cow's milk products temporarily from your diet – and see if this helps your baby. It may be a good idea to discuss this plan first with your health visitor or GP.

Avoiding all milk products is difficult. Milk is used in various forms in many manufactured foods. Apart from cutting out all dairy products, you will also have to avoid most margarines, some breakfast cereals, biscuits and crisps, and many other foods. Look carefully at food labels. You will have to avoid milk for two weeks. If, after this time, you feel that your baby's colic is definitely better and you decide to carry on with a milk-free diet, ask to be referred to a dietitian. She will give you expert advice on eating a nutritious diet without milk, and will also help you decide for how long you need to avoid milk.

Breastfeeding and allergies

Breastfeeding helps to protect against allergies. All babies tend to be short of a special chemical called IgA, but babies in allergic families have particularly low levels. Breastmilk is rich in IgA. Drinking breastmilk also encourages the baby's own body to make more IgA.

This protection is best if your baby is given nothing but breastmilk for the first six months. Some experts feel that even a single bottle of artificial baby milk during this time may allow allergies to develop.

There is some research evidence that this protection can be increased by changes to the breastfeeding mother's diet. Two research studies found that when mothers in allergic families did not eat foods such as eggs, dairy products and nuts, their breastfed babies were less likely to develop allergic conditions while they were very young. (The protection became weaker as they got older.)

If you (or your baby's father) have allergic problems, it may be a good idea to discuss these ideas with your doctor. If you decide to restrict what you eat while breast-feeding, you will need expert dietary advice to help prevent shortages of important nutrients.

Key points

❏ Breastmilk will give your baby health benefits that will stay with her throughout her life. A good supply of breastmilk depends on feeding your baby when she wants to feed, and making sure that she is well attached to your breast. Learning any new skill can be hard. Loving support and sound information will make learning to breastfeed easier.

❏ Eat to appetite whilst breastfeeding. Many women settle into a routine of four meals a day, and a snack in the middle of the night. Drink whenever you are thirsty.

❏ Women who eat a vegan diet may need a supplement of vitamin B_{12}. Some women may benefit from a supplement of calcium – women breastfeeding twins, very young women, and women who do not like dairy produce and other foods rich in calcium. Other women may need a supplement of vitamin D – women who do not expose their skin to the sun in summer, or who do not like foods rich in vitamin D.

❏ Always tell your doctor, dentist or pharmacist that you are breastfeeding. Avoid aspirin in any form.

❏ The birth of your baby is a good time to stop smoking. If you smoke, your baby breathes in your smoke as well as taking in poisons through your milk. Breastfed babies of smokers tend to cry more than do other babies. Regular use of cannabis whilst breastfeeding may be extremely harmful. Get help soon. Drinking more than 6 units of alcohol a day whilst breastfeeding may slow your baby's motor development. Light drinking – 1 unit of alcohol or less each day – probably does no harm.

❏ Certain foods eaten by mothers may cause colic in their babies – but this has not yet been proven by research. Eat a full and varied diet, unless you feel sure that a particular food is disturbing your baby. Smoking, and too much caffeine, both seem to cause colic in some babies. Very occasionally, colic may be caused by a baby's reaction to cow's milk protein in her mother's diet.

❏ Breastfeeding protects against allergies. This protection is best if your baby is given nothing but breast-milk for her first six months.

❏ You don't need to avoid mould-ripened cheeses such as Brie, Stilton or Camembert when you are breast-feeding but still avoid predatory fish including sword-fish, shark and more than one fresh tuna steak or two medium tins a week.

About the
National Childbirth Trust

Run by parents, for parents, the National Childbirth Trust is a self-help support charity with 350 branches across the UK. There's bound to be a local branch near you, running:

- ❑ childbirth classes
- ❑ breastfeeding counselling
- ❑ new baby groups
- ❑ open house get-togethers
- ❑ support for dads
- ❑ working parents' groups
- ❑ nearly new sales of baby clothes and equipment

– as well as loads of events where you can meet and make friends with other people going through the same changes.

- To find the contact details of your nearest branch, ring the NCT Enquiry Line: 0870 444 8707 or log on to: www.nctpregnancyandbabycare.com
- To find answers to pregnancy queries, you can also contact the Enquiry Line or website above.
- To speak to a breastfeeding counsellor, ring the NCT Breastfeeding Line: 0870 444 8708.
- To buy excellent baby goods, maternity bras and gifts, visit: www.nctms.co.uk or telephone 0870 112 1120.
- To join the NCT with a debit or credit card, just call 0870 990 8040.

You don't have to become a member to enjoy the services and support of the National Childbirth Trust. It's open to everyone. We do encourage people to join the charity because it helps fund our work – supporting all parents.

When you become an NCT member and join your local group, you'll get a regular neighbourhood newsletter (a guide to the area aimed at new parents) and you'll also receive NCT's *New Generation* – our mailed out members' magazine that takes an in-depth look at all issues of interest to new parents.

'*The NCT support network is second to none. It's very reassuring and comforting.*'

The National Childbirth Trust wants all parents to have an experience of pregnancy, birth and early parenthood that enriches their lives and gives them confidence in being a parent.

National Childbirth Trust, Alexandra House, Oldham Terrace, London W3 6NH. Tel: 0870 770 3236

Useful organisations

Sainsbury's/WellBeing 'Eating for Pregnancy' telephone helpline: 0845 130 3646 (local call rate)

Research-based advice on nutrition for women before, during and after pregnancy.

Food Standards Agency
Aviation House
125 Kingsway
London
WC2B 6NH
Tel: 020 7276 8000
www.foodstandards.gov.uk
A government food safety watchdog, publicising safe eating and promoting good nutrition.

The Food Commission
94 White Lion Street
London N1 9PF
Tel: 020 7837 2250
www.foodcomm.org.uk
An independent watchdog on food issues.

Vegetarian Society
Parkdale
Dunham Road
Altrincham
Cheshire WA14 4QG
Tel: 0161 925 2000
www.vegsoc.org.uk

Vegan Society
Donald Watson House
7 Battle Road
St Leonard's on Sea
East Sussex TN37 7AA
Tel: 0845 45 88244 (local rate)
www.vegansociety.com

Toxoplasmosis Trust
Room 26, 61-71 Collier Street
London N1 9BE
Tel: 0870 777 3060
Helpline: 020 7593 1149 (9am–5pm weekdays)
Support and up-to-date information for sufferers of toxo-
plasmosis and their families.

Pregnancy and parenting

Action on Pre-eclampsia (APEC)
84-88 Pinner Road
Harrow
Middlesex HA1 4HZ
Helpline: 020 8427 4217 (10am-1pm weekdays)
www.apec.org.uk
Support for sufferers and information for public and health professionals.

Association for Spina Bifida and Hydrocephalus (ASBAH)
ASBAH House
42 Park Road
Peterborough PE1 2UQ
Tel: 01733 555988
Support for affected families, and information about the conditions, including the use of folic acid during pregnancy.

Twins and Multiple Births Association (TAMBA)
2 The Willows
Gardner Road
Guildford
Surrey GU1 4PG
Helpline: 01732 868000 (7pm-11pm weekdays, 10am-11pm weekends)
www.tamba.org.uk
Encouragement and support, nationally and locally, for parents of twins, triplets or more.

Disabled Parents Network
Parent-to-parent support: 0870 241 0450
www.disabledparentsnetwork.org.uk

Foresight
28 The Paddock
Godalming
Surrey GU7 1XD
Tel: 01483 427839
www.foresight-preconception.org.uk
Advice on pre-conceptual care for both parents, with emphasis on nutritional analyses and supplementation.

Medical conditions

Diabetes UK
10 Parkway
London NW1 7AA
Tel: 020 7424 1000
www.diabetes.org.uk

Coeliac Society
PO Box 220
High Wycombe
Bucks HP11 2HY
Tel: 01494 437278
www.coeliac.co.uk

Eating Disorders Association (EDA)
103 Prince of Wales Road
Norwich
Norfolk NR1 1DW
Helpline: 0845 634 1414 (8.30am–10.30pm weekdays)
Youth helpline: 0845 634 7650 (4pm–6.30pm weekdays)
www.edauk.com
Information and help on all aspects of eating disorders.

Allergy

Anaphylaxis Campaign
PO Box 149
Fleet
Hants GU13 9XU
Tel: 01252 542029
www.anaphylaxis.org.uk
Support for sufferers and guidance for public and health professionals on potentially fatal allergies, such as peanut allergy.

Allergy UK
Deepdene House
30 Bellegrove Road
Welling, Kent DA16 3PY
Helpline: 020 8303 8583 (9am–9pm weekdays, 10am–1pm Saturdays)
www.allergyfoundation.com
Information packs tailored to individual needs.

Smoking, alcohol and drug abuse

Quitline (helping smokers to cut down or stop)
0800 002200
Pregnancy Quitline 0800 002211
Drinkline (helping drinkers to cut down)
0800 917 8282
National drugs helpline: 0800 776600 (freephone)

Action on Smoking and Health (ASH)
102 Clifton Street
London EC2A 4HW
Tel: 020 7739 5902
www.ash.org.uk
A campaigning public health charity working towards the elimination of tobacco use.

Alcohol Concern
Waterbridge House
32–36 Loman Street
London SE1 0EE
Tel: 020 7922 8699
www.alcoholconcern.org.uk
Information and resources.

Index